ZWEITES INTERNATIONALES SYMPOSIUM ÜBER NEUROSEKRETION

LUND VOM 1. BIS 6. JULI 1957

HERAUSGEGEBEN VON

W. BARGMANN · KIEL **B. HANSTRÖM** · LUND
B. UND **E. SCHARRER** · NEW YORK

MIT 71 ABBILDUNGEN
DAVON 2 FARBIG

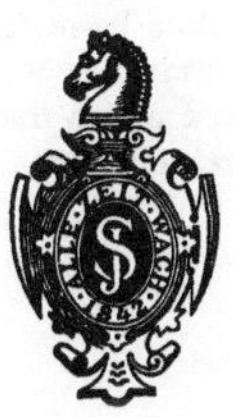

SPRINGER-VERLAG
BERLIN · GÖTTINGEN · HEIDELBERG
1958

ISBN 978-3-642-53253-5   ISBN 978-3-642-53252-8 (eBook)
DOI 10.1007/978-3-642-53252-8

Preface

In recent years investigation of the phenomenon of neurosecretion has proceeded largely along lines that emerged from the discussions of the first Symposium on Neurosecretion, held at the Zoological Station, Naples, Italy, in 1953 [Pubbl. Staz. Zool. **24,** Suppl. 1—98 (1954)].

New insights were gained as a result of the use of the electron microscope. Considerable progress was made in the chemical analysis of the material produced and released by neurosecretory cells. The rôle of neurosecretory centers in the neuroendocrine control of various physiological functions in invertebrates and vertebrates is understood a great deal better today than a few years ago. These and related topics were discussed at the Second Symposium on Neurosecretion, held at the University of Lund, Sweden, July 1—6, 1957. As in the case of the Proceedings of the Naples Symposium the manuscripts of the formal papers were collected by the editors some time after the meeting in order to enable the authors to include the essentials of the discussions which followed each paper. To record the discussions verbatim seemed less important than to risk the loss of spontaneity which might result from the presence of recording apparatus.

The organization of such a meeting requires the dedicated cooperation of many persons and the good will of various agencies. The members of the Symposium were unanimous in their praise and gratitude for their gracious hosts at Lund. The Rockefeller Foundation generously contributed a fund of 4000.- Sw.-Crowns toward the expenses.

A number of participants received travel subsidies from organizations in their respective countries. The splendid cooperation of the Springer Verlag in making possible the publication of the proceedings of the symposium is here gratefully acknowledged. Thus the Second Symposium on Neurosecretion owed whatever it accomplished to a large measure of active support on the part of many individuals and agencies.

W. BARGMANN   B. HANSTRÖM

E. and B. SCHARRER

Inhaltsverzeichnis

(der Vortragsfolge entsprechend)

Der vorliegende Band enthält die Mehrzahl der zum Vortrage auf dem Zweiten Symposium über Neurosekretion in Lund angemeldeten Mitteilungen, denen eine Begrüßungsansprache des Rector Magnificus Professor PHILIP SANDBLOM voranging. Die Titel von Vorträgen, deren Manuskripte nicht eingingen, sind durch * gekennzeichnet. Von einer Wiedergabe der ausgiebigen Diskussionen wurde abgesehen.

Inhaltsverzeichnis

V

Introduction

By

BERTIL HANSTRÖM

Volume 24 (Supplemento) of the Pubblicazioni della Stazione Zoologica di Napoli 1954, which contains the proceedings of the First Symposium on Neurosecretion, organized by ERNST and BERTA SCHARRER and held in Naples May 11—18th, 1953, ends with the following words:

"The coming years will certainly bring new observations and insights, be it in the direction indicated above (i. e. the "Summary of the Symposium") or along other lines. In some years hence we may again be wondering where we stand and what progress we have made; we shall then meet at Lund, Sweden."

Thus I was charged with the task of arranging the *Second Symposium on Neurosecretion*. This I could not have managed without the valuable help of several friends and colleagues, and foremost ERNST and BERTA SCHARRER, New York, and WOLFGANG BARGMANN, Kiel, supported by ELLEN and MATHIAS THOMSEN and K. G. WINGSTRAND, Copenhagen. Through grants from the Swedish government and the Rockefeller Foundation it was possible to reduce the participants' living expenses during their stay in Lund and on the last day, to arrange a general excursion to the nature sanctuary of Kullen in northwestern Scania.

Through the courtesy of Professor GEORG KAHLSON and Dr. med. DORA JACOBSOHN the Symposium could be held at the modern Physiological Institute. The proceedings started with an address of welcome given by the Rector of the University of Lund, PHILIP SANDBLOM, Professor of Surgery. This was followed by my opening address, which is summarized in the following section.

Mr. Vice-chancellor, dear Colleagues and Friends:

I should like to repeat Professor SANDBLOM's words of welcome to a town which, founded by King Canute the Great, in the springtime of Scandinavian culture had important international relations in spite of its small size. The kingdom of Canute comprised not only Denmark, to which this present southern province of Sweden then belonged, but also Norway and England, and in 1103 Lund was the seat of the archbishop of Scandinavia, who was the spiritual head of Denmark, Sweden, Norway, Iceland and Greenland. Perhaps I should also mention the fact that the cathedral in Lund, started in 1085, is the oldest remaining building in Scandinavia and that the Cathedral School has the oldest traditions of any educational establishment in this part of Europe; it started its activity in the year 1100.

The second symposium on neurosecretion is held in this country in the year 1957, which marks the 250th anniversary of the birth of CARL LINNAEUS, an anniversary which has recently been commemorated in Sweden, Great Britain,

France, the Netherlands, and several other countries. It is true that LINNAEUS belongs first and foremost to Uppsala, but he spent his first student year in Lund, and he seems to have received important help and stimulation from his teacher here, Professor ANDREAS STOBAEUS. There are two Swedish scientists of the eighteenth century in whose memory special houses of honour have been built in London, CARL LINNAEUS and EMANUEL SWEDENBORG. The first of these buildings is the well known Burlington House, the second is simply called the Swedenborg House. As a professor at Uppsala while actively teaching medicine, LINNAEUS never mentioned anything which could be interpreted even as a glimpse of a secretory function of the nervous system, whereas Swedenborg, as emphasized by Professor Sir SOLLY ZUCKERMAN, had accepted and further elaborated the old conception of a lymph which was produced by the brain to be collected into the hypophysis and released into the jugular veins. Swedenborg finally exchanged his studies in natural science for religious meditations and, just 200 years ago, in 1757, founded a church, the new Jerusalem. There is, however, another anniversary of which I want to remind you on this occasion, the three hundred years anniversary of the death of the Englishman WILLIAM HARVEY, perhaps the greatest of all medical scientists. His discovery of the circulation of the blood ought to be remembered in connection with proceedings dealing with neurosecretion and thus with substances which, like the secretions of the brain according to Swedenborg, "imbue the blood with its own inmost essence, nature and life" and for which the circulation of blood is necessary in order that the secretions shall be able to fulfil their mission.

Since the last time we met, the number of contributions to the subject of neurosecretion has rapidly increased. It is quite impossible to mention more than a few names of authors and a small number of new facts which have been published during these four years. And when, in addition to the general surveys of the neurosecretory phenomenon which have been edited during this period by ERNST and BERTA SCHARRER, WOLFGANG BARGMANN and others, I mention certain details, this must be understood as an expression of my own private interests and views. Thus I remind you of the Nobel prize for the analysis and synthesis of the posterior lobe hormones of the hypophysis received by VINCENT DU VIGNEAUD, who was assisted by a large group of able biochemists, among them H. B. VAN DYKE, of other biochemical investigations by A. BUTENANDT and P. KARLSON on the substances from the endocrine system of the insect head, by J. C. SLOPER on the occurrence of protein-bound cystine in the neurosecretory substance not only in the hypothalamus of vertebrates but also in the corpora cardiaca of insects, and of the chemical nature of the colour change hormone in crustaceans and insects by the intimate cooperation of several scientists in England, France, Italy and Sweden. The interesting similarities in structure and composition of the neurosecretory systems of insects and crustaceans have been still more accentuated by the discovery of the Y-organ in the latter by M. GABE, who has also contributed to the understanding of the neurosecretory systems in chilopods and diplopods, while the latest papers by M. ENAMI and K. IMAI have displayed an astonishing parallel development in the anatomy and histology of the neurohypophysis of the head and the so-called neurohypophysis spinalis at the caudal end of the spinal cord in fishes. In this connection a welcome contribution to the morphological and physiological parallelism between the neuro-secretory systems of insects and vertebrates would be the verification of a hormonal control of the function of the anterior lobe of the hypophysis by the hypothalamic neurosecretory system, of which we hope to hear more during the course of this symposium. This subject has recently been excellently treated by for instance G. W. HARRIS in his "Neural control of the pituitary gland" and from a different viewpoint by J. BENOIT and I. ASSENMACHER and by L. MARTINI.

J. H. WELSH, chiefly on account of his investigations of hormones which regulate the function of the heart in molluscs (supported by D. BLISS in her studies of the metabolism, regeneration and growth of crabs), has inferred that neurohormones may be divided into neurohumors like acetylcholine, adrenaline and noradrenaline, which act mostly at short range and for relatively brief durations, and neurosecretory substances which may act at some distance from the point of release and for relatively long periods of time.

The important physiological role which substances produced by nerve cells evidently play according to the investigations of the last 15 years has caused R. B. CLARK to present a hypothesis that neurosecretory cells are more primitive than ordinary nerve cells which are only concerned with the propagation of impulses. I agree with CLARK insofar as the production of the substances which WELSH calls neurohumors probably must be as old as and a necessary foundation for the transmission of nervous impulses. But I must retain the view that the separation of the nervous system from the epithelium occurred in order to form an organ primarily for conducting impulses and not for the production of secretions.

Finally, a very important contribution to the knowledge of the true nature of the neurosecretory cells are the observations by D. D. POTTER and O. LOEWEN-STEIN that these cells are capable of receiving and conducting nerve impulses even though they actively produce and transport a considerable amount of neurosecretory matter. The study of neurosecretion evidently has now passed its juvenile revolutionary stage and is "coming of age".

Aus der Elektronenmikroskopischen Abteilung am Anatomischen Institut der Universität Kiel
(Direktor: Prof. Dr. W. Bargmann)

Elektronenmikroskopische Untersuchungen an der Neurohypophyse

Von

W. Bargmann

Mit 6 Abbildungen

Die Zahl der elektronenmikroskopischen Studien, die sich mit der Struktur des neurosekretorischen Zwischenhirn-Hypophysensystems beschäftigen, ist noch verhältnismäßig gering. Als erster hat es Schiebler (1952) unternommen, das Neurosekret aus dem Hypophysenhinterlappen des Rindes durch Differentialzentrifugieren zu gewinnen und die so erhaltene granuläre Fraktion, deren Körnchen sich mit Chromalaunhämatoxylin färben, elektronenoptisch zu analysieren. Nach den bisher vorliegenden Erfahrungen ist allerdings damit zu rechnen, daß die Methode des Zentrifugierens granuläre Partikel liefert, denen intracytoplasmatische Granula gleicher Beschaffenheit im Ausgangsmaterial nicht entsprechen; es sei nur kurz auf die Mikrosomen-Problematik hingewiesen. Es fragt sich daher, ob die von Schiebler beschriebenen Granula mit einem Durchmesser von 0,5—2,5 μ nicht ein Gemenge von Neurosekretgranula, deren Fragmenten und denen anderer Zellbestandteile darstellen. Ein den Cytologen befriedigender Weg zur Aufdeckung der Feinstruktur neurosekretorischer Elemente eröffnete sich erst nach der Einführung der Schnittmethode in die Elektronenmikroskopie.

Elektronenmikroskopische Untersuchungen an Feinschnitten verdanken wir Palay (1955, 1957), Green und van Breemen (1955), Duncan (1956) und Fujita (1957). Sie legen neben neuen Befunden neue Fragen vor.

Zunächst ist hervorzuheben, daß meines Wissens keine neuere Arbeit das morphologische Verhalten der *Perikaryen* neurosekretorischer Neurone zum Gegenstand hat, wenn man von kurzen Hinweisen Palays absieht. Hier liegt also noch Neuland der Forschung vor. Aus den Mitteilungen über die *Endstation* der neurosekretorischen Bahn, d. h. über die Endigungen ihrer marklosen Fasern im Hinterlappen, ist folgendes ersichtlich: Die Nervenendigungen im Hinterlappen der Ratte enthalten außer Mitochondrien die bekannten "synaptic vesicles" [Durchmesser 230—300 Å (Palay)] und als charakteristische Bildungen Granula bzw. "vesicles" mit einem Durchmesser von 100—150 mμ. Die Mehrzahl dieser Gebilde ist mit einem dichten zentralen Körperchen ausgestattet, das durch eine hellere Zone von einer oberflächlichen Membran getrennt ist. Daneben kommen elektronenoptisch leere Bläschen gleicher Größenordnung vor. Bei dehydrierten Tieren, d. h. solchen, denen eine 2,5%ige Salzlösung als Trinkflüssigkeit über 6—13 Tage verabfolgt wurde, überwiegen diese leeren "vesicles".

Palay ist der Auffassung, die mit dichten Zentren ausgestatteten Granula entsprächen den mit Chromalaunhämatoxylin elektiv färbbaren, lichtmikroskopisch sichtbaren Neurosekretkörnchen. Die gleichen Granula kommen nach seinen Angaben im Perikaryon und in den gröberen Fortsätzen der Neurone des Nucleus supraopticus vor. Auch auf den methodisch weniger befriedigenden, im Jahre 1955 veröffentlichten elektronenmikroskopischen Aufnahmen der Neurohypophyse von Säugern, die Green und van Breemen vorlegen, erkennt man zahlreiche osmiophile Körnchen, über deren Lagerung im Axoplasma oder im Cytoplasma von Gliazellen sich die Autoren jedoch nicht entschieden äußern. Ferner bildet Fujita (1957) elektronenmikroskopische Aufnahmen aus dem Hinterlappen der Hundehypophyse ab, auf denen man kugelige Körnchen mit einem Durchmesser von 100—300 mμ im Inneren von Faserdurchschnitten wahrnimmt. Auch Fujita ist der Meinung, diese Granula seien Neurosekretkörnchen. Schließlich sind Duncans (1955, 1956) Untersuchungen an der Neurohypophyse des Hühnchens zu erwähnen, in denen über Neurosekretgranula von hoher Dichte (Durchmesser 0,1—0,2 μ) im Inneren von Nervenfasern berichtet wird. Der größte Teil dieser Körnchen erscheint homogen, einige weisen eine zentrale Aufhellung auf.

Überblickt man die genannten Veröffentlichungen, so stößt man zunächst auf eine Differenz zwischen den Angaben Fujitas und der übrigen Autoren hinsichtlich der Abgrenzung der marklosen Nervenfasern im Hinterlappen. Fujita spricht nämlich von einer im übrigen Schrifttum nicht erwähnten Doppelmembran, welche die Fasern gegen die Umgebung abgrenzen soll. Es erscheint daher notwendig, diese Angabe nachzuprüfen, wenngleich Fujitas Abbildungen Einzelheiten nicht mit hinlänglicher Deutlichkeit wiedergeben. Man muß weiter anstreben, auf Längsschnitten durch marklose Fasern des Hinterlappens, deren bildliche Darstellung noch aussteht, die tatsächliche Zugehörigkeit der Granula enthaltenden Areale zu Nervenfasern überzeugend darzutun. Berechtigt ist ferner der Wunsch, die lichtmikroskopisch begründete Vorstellung von der strukturellen Einheitlichkeit des neurosekretorischen Systems in der Wirbeltierreihe durch elektronenoptische Studien an Vertretern anderer Wirbeltierklassen zu erhärten; bisher liegen lediglich elektronenmikroskopische Arbeiten über das Gefüge des Hinterlappens von Säugern und Vögeln vor. Schließlich fragt es sich, ob die elektronenmikroskopisch darstellbaren Granula wirklich dem lichtmikroskopisch in Form von Granula faßbaren Neurosekret entsprechen.

Bevor wir uns diesen Fragen anhand neuer Beobachtungen zuwenden, seien noch die in den zitierten Veröffentlichungen enthaltenen Angaben über die *Pituicyten* kurz beleuchtet, denen eine Beteiligung an den neurosekretorischen Vorgängen im Hinterlappen zugeschrieben wird. Lichtmikroskopisch ließ sich bisher nicht völlig sicher entscheiden, ob Neurosekretgranula im Cytoplasma der Gliazellen des Hinterlappens vorkommen oder nicht. Green und van Breemen (1955) äußern sich über die Lokalisation der Körnchen auf Grund ihrer elektronenoptischen Untersuchungen — wie schon erwähnt — zurückhaltend. Palays (1955, 1957) Schilderung enthält keine Angaben über das Vorkommen von Neurosekretgranula in den Pituicyten. Nach seinen Ausführungen kann man die Ausläufer dieser Zellen von den Nervenfasern, die sich eng an sie anschmiegen, unterscheiden, da erstere Lipoidtröpfchen und feine Granula (Durchmesser 150 Å)

aufweisen, die den von Palade beschriebenen Granula des basophilen Cyto-
plasmas ähneln. Da Palays Aussage noch vereinzelt dasteht, ist es angezeigt,
die Struktur der Pituicyten in weiteren elektronenmikroskopischen Untersuchungen zu studieren. Dabei soll auf die Beziehungen dieser Zellen nicht nur
zu den Nervenfasern, sondern auch zu den Kapillarwänden geachtet werden.

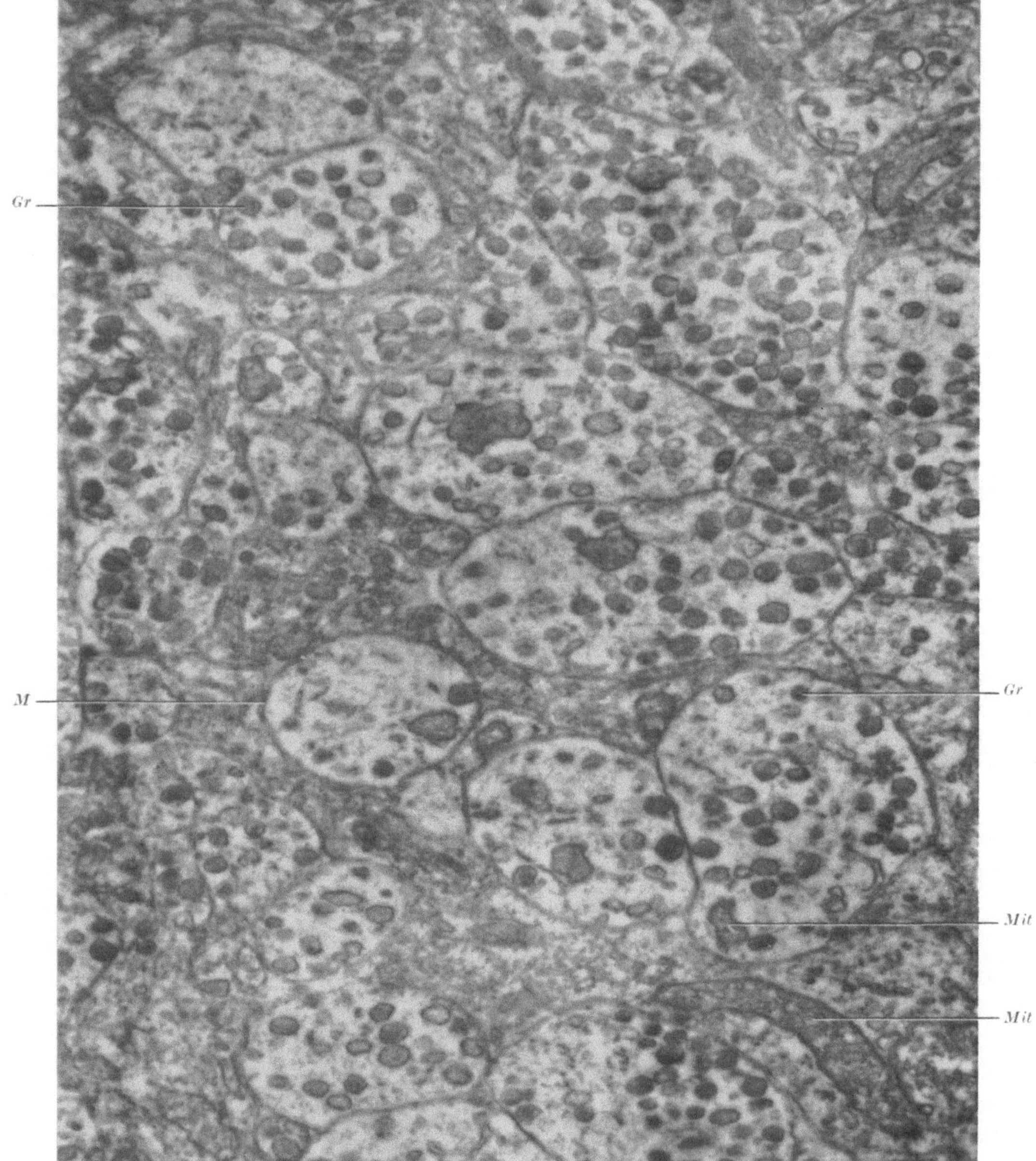

Abb. 1. Hinterlappen der Katze (elektronenopt. Vergr. 6800fach, Gesamtvergr. 27 000fach). *M* Membran markloser
Nervenfaser. *Mit* Mitochondrien, *Gr* Granula innerhalb der Nervenfasern. Aus Bargmann und Knoop (1957)

Unsere eigenen elektronenmikroskopischen Untersuchungen erstrecken sich auf die Neurohypophyse von Säugern [Katze, Hund, BARGMANN und KNOOP

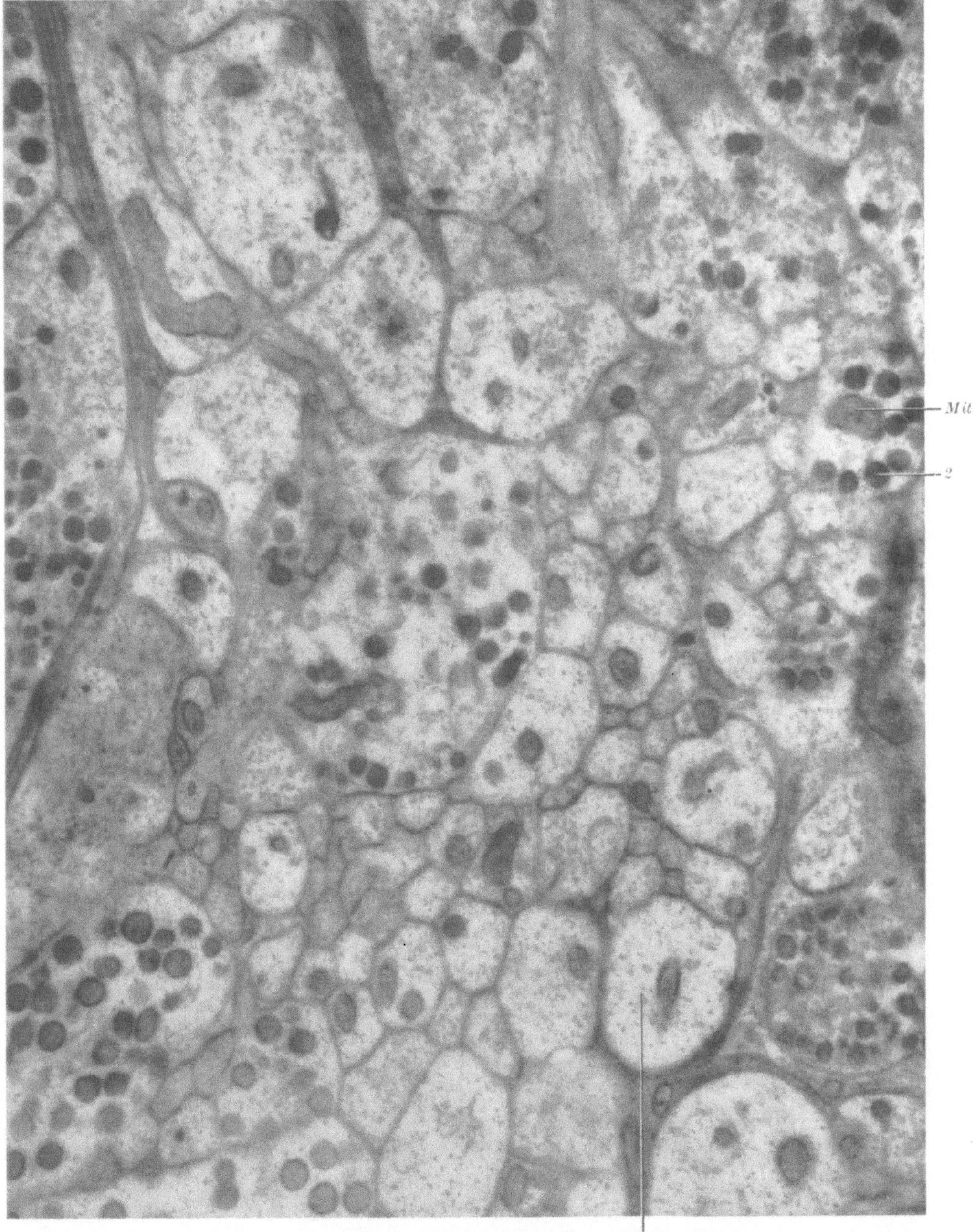

Abb. 2. Hinterlappen von Tropidonotus natrix mit quergetroffenen marklosen Nervenfasern, deren Neuroplasma teils nur Mitochondrien enthält (1), teils mehr oder weniger zahlreiche Granula (2). *Mit* Mitochondrien. (Vergr. 33000fach, zur Reproduktion verkl.). Aus BARGMANN, KNOOP und THIEL (1957)

(1957), s. dort Methodik], ferner von Reptilien (Anguis, Tropidonotus). Teils in Bestätigung, teils in Erweiterung der Angaben der oben genannten Autoren wurden folgende Befunde erhoben: In Präparaten des Hinterlappens erkennt man in dichter Fügung die Anschnitte rundlicher Gebilde, die von einer zarten

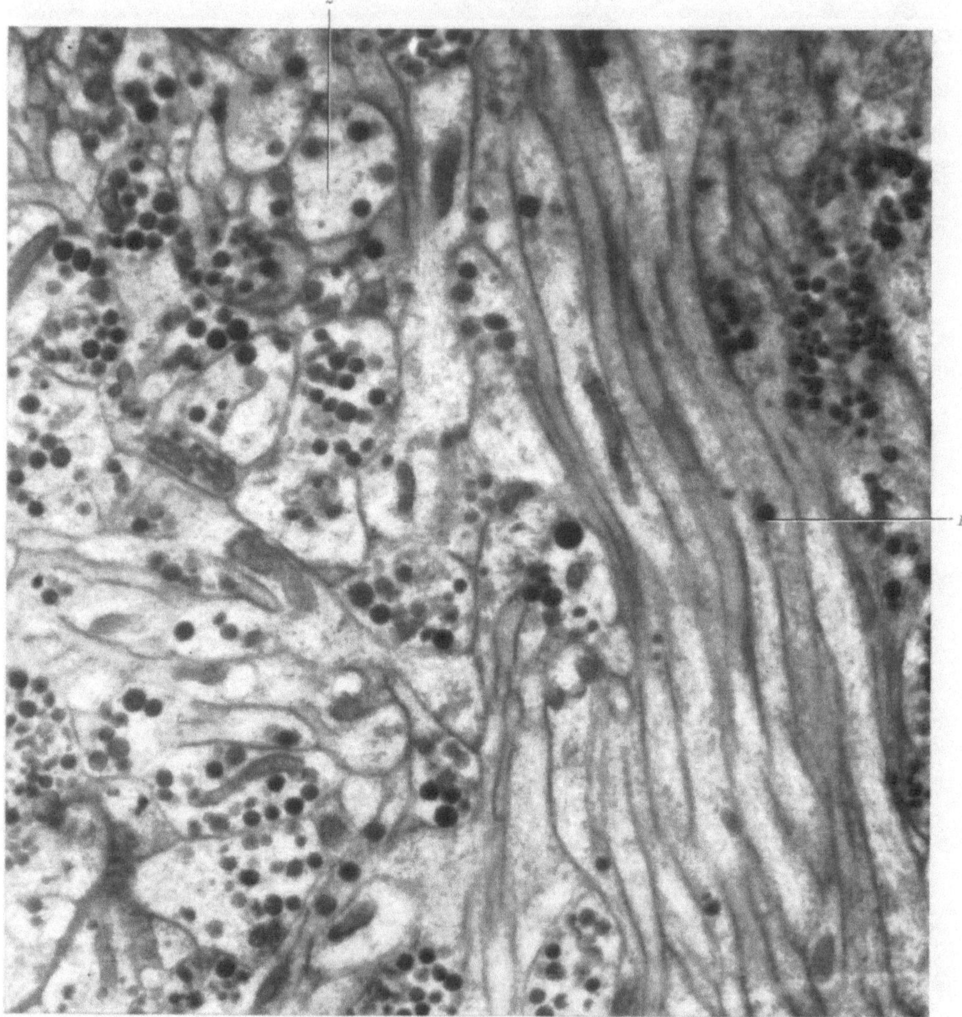

Abb. 3. Längs- und quergetroffene marklose Nervenfasern im Hinterlappen von Tropidonotus natrix. *1* Granulum in längsgetroffener Faser, *2* quergetroffene Faser mit 4 Granula. (Vergr. 15500fach, zur Reproduktion verkl.). Aus BARGMANN, KNOOP und THIEL (1957)

Membran begrenzt werden, d. h. nicht von einer Doppelmembran im Sinne FUJITAs. Diese Gebilde schließen außer Mitochondrien "synaptic vesicles", parallelisierte Filamente und Granula besonderer Art ein. Die naheliegende Annahme, es handele sich um Durchschnitte durch marklose Nervenfasern bzw. deren Anschwellungen, wird durch Aufnahmen bestätigt, auf denen kürzere oder längere Strecken von Fasern mit den granulahaltigen Auftreibungen in Kontinuität zu erkennen sind [Abb. bei Bargmann und Knoop (1957)]. Hinzu kommt die Tatsache, daß die erwähnten Granula besonderer Art auch in längsgetroffenen Faserabschnitten sichtbar sind (Abb. 3).

Die Durchmesser der kugeligen Granula betragen bei der Katze 1200—1800 Å, bei Tropidonotus 1500—3000 Å. Es erscheint bemerkenswert, daß an Körnchen reiche, aufgetriebene Faserpartien mehr Mitochondrien enthalten als körnchenarme Faserstrecken. Die Struktur der Granula stimmt bei Säugern und Reptilien überein. Sie werden von einer dünnen Membran umschlossen, während ihr Inneres eine dichte Substanz enthält, die vielfach durch eine schmale, hellere

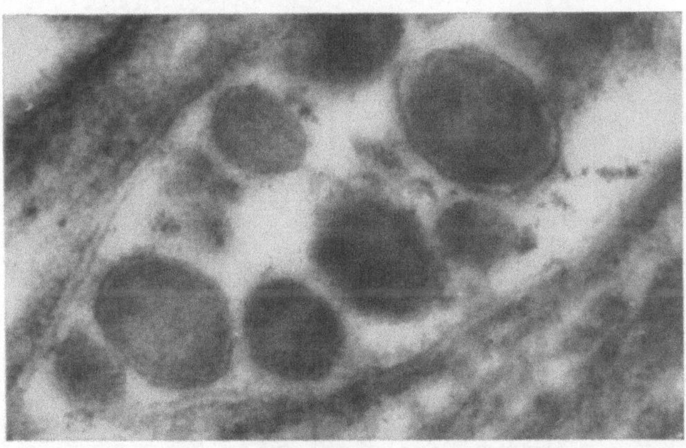

Abb. 4. Granula im Neuroplasma einer neurosekretorischen Faser im Hinterlappen von Tropidonotus natrix. Beachte die Körnchenmembran. (Vergr. 110000fach). Aus Bargmann, Knoop und Thiel (1957)

Zone von der Membran geschieden ist (Abb. 4). Ferner kommen, jedoch in geringerer Zahl, optisch leere, bläschenartige Gebilde vor, wie sie Palay unter experimentellen Bedingungen beobachtet hat.

Da diese Granula eine Besonderheit der Nervenfasern des Hinterlappens darstellen, erscheint es erlaubt, daß man in ihnen das Substrat des färberisch darstellbaren Neurosekrets vermutet. Diese Granula sind mit den angegebenen Werten ihrer Durchmesser z. T. beträchtlich kleiner als Mitochondrien, so daß mit einer lichtmikroskopischen Sichtbarkeit jedes einzelnen Granulums nicht zu rechnen ist. Daher ist anzunehmen, daß das im lichtmikroskopischen Präparat gerade eben erkennbare Neurosekretgranulum einer Körnchenballung entspricht, von gut sichtbaren gröberen Tröpfchen ganz zu schweigen.

Eine Bestätigung dieser Auffassung erbringen Befunde, die erst nach dem Symposium gewonnen werden konnten [Bargmann, Knoop und Thiel (1957)]; es ist sinnvoll, an dieser Stelle im Nachtrag auf sie zu verweisen. Wie Abb. 5 erkennen läßt, stellen größere, lichtmikroskopisch darstellbare Neurosekretpartikel jeweils ein *Aggregat* miteinander versinterter Granula (Elementargranula) dar, deren Konturen auf Schnitten durch derartige Tröpfchen (Durchmesser 17000—22000 Å) als helle Linien hervortreten. Bisher ergaben sich keine Hinweise auf die Art der Entstehung dieser Elementar- oder Primärgranula. Vielleicht wird man bezüglich dieses Problems klarer sehen können, wenn ausgiebigere elektronenmikroskopische Untersuchungen am Perikaryon der neurosekretorischen Zellen vorliegen, in denen die Mehrzahl der Neurosekretionsforscher auf Grund lichtoptischer Feststellungen den Bildungsort des Neurosekrets erblickt.

Die unregelmäßig gestalteten, mit Ausläufern versehenen Leiber der *Pituicyten* enthalten bald ovoide, bald zerklüftete Zellkerne, zahlreiche, z. T. große Mito-

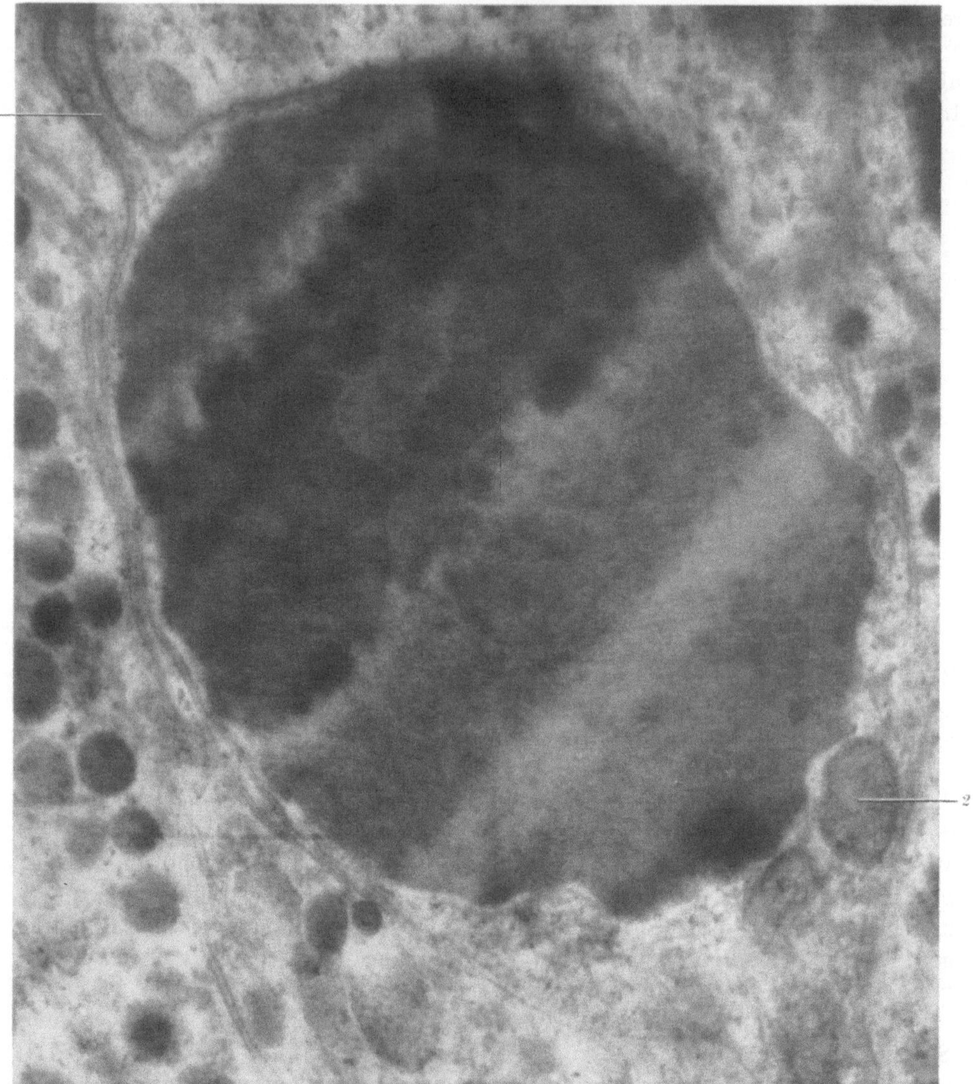

Abb. 5. Neurosekrettropfen im Hinterlappen von Tropidonotus natrix, in einer Anschwellung einer marklosen Nervenfaser. Der Tropfen besteht aus einem Aggregat von Granula, deren Umrisse noch erkennbar sind. *1* dünner Faserabschnitt, *2* Mitochondrion. (Vergr. 73 000fach, zur Reproduktion verkl.).
Aus Bargmann, Knoop und Thiel (1957)

chondrien, endoplasmatisches Reticulum sowie vereinzelte homogen erscheinende Granula, die jedoch nicht mit den geschilderten Neurosekretkörnchen identisch sind. Zwischen dem Perikaryon der Pituicyten und den sekrethaltigen Nerven-

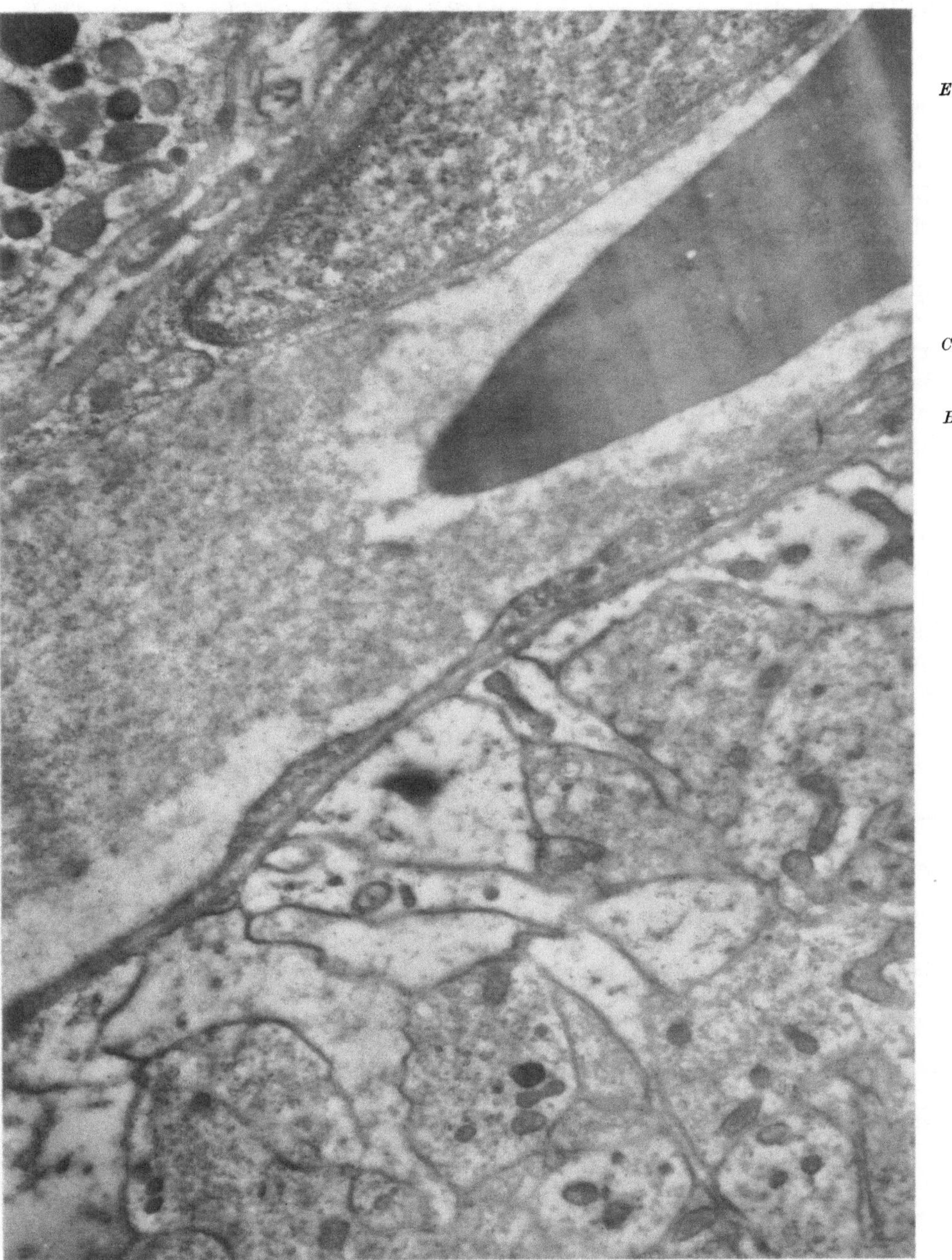

Abb. 6. Blutcapillare an der Grenze von Hinter- und Zwischenlappen in der Hypophyse von Tropidonotus natrix. *E* Endothelkern, *Er* Erythrocytenanschnitt, *B* Basalmembran, *C* Cytoplasmaschicht des Endothels. Beachte strukturarme und an „vesicles" reiche Nervenfaserendigungen, die sich der Basalmembran anschmiegen (untere Bildhälfte). (Vergr. 30000fach, zur Reproduktion verkl.)

fasern bestehen insofern enge Beziehungen, als die Nervenfasern in Auskehlungen des Pituicytenleibes eingebettet sind, so daß der Abstand zwischen Kernoberfläche des Pituicyten und Oberfläche der Fasern stellenweise nur gering ist.

Nervenfasern und wahrscheinlich auch die Ausläufer von Pituicyten erreichen die Oberfläche der *Blutcapillaren*, deren Basalmembran (Abb. 6) sie sich innig anschmiegen. In der Neurohypophyse von Tropidonotus findet man auf der Außenfläche der Capillaren teils kolbige Verdickungen unbestreitbar von Nervenfasern, Mitochondrien, "synaptic vesicles" und Sekretgranula enthaltend, teils strukturarme Cytoplasmaformationen, in denen außer einzelnen Mitochondrien nur spärliche Bläschen und verwaschene Gerinnselstrukturen sichtbar sind. Während es sich im letzteren Falle um entweder sekretfreie oder präparativ veränderte Nervenendigungen handeln dürfte, mögen auffallend dünne lamellenartige Strukturen blattartigen Fortsätzen von Pituicyten angehören. Eine poröse Bauweise des Capillarendothels (Palay), das stellenweise nur 300 Å dick ist, wurde von uns bei Säugern bisher nicht beobachtet. Lediglich bei Tropidonotus fanden wir eine einzelne Lücke in der auf weite Strecken hin geschlossenen Endothelschicht.

Die hier auf Grund fremder und eigener Beobachtungen mitgeteilten Befunde über das strukturelle Verhalten der Neurohypophyse der Wirbeltiere befinden sich mit den auf lichtmikroskopische Erfahrungen sich stützenden Angaben über den Feinbau neurosekretorischer Elemente in guter Übereinstimmung. Es bleibt abzuwarten, ob diese Beobachtungen mit den Aussagen elektronenoptischer Studien an neurosekretorischen Systemen von Wirbellosen grundsätzlich in Einklang stehen.

Literatur

Bargmann, W., u. A. Knoop: Elektronenmikroskopische Beobachtungen an der Neurohypophyse. Z. Zellforsch. **46**, 242—251 (1957).

— — u. A. Thiel: Elektronenmikroskopische Studie an der Neurohypophyse von *Tropidonotus natrix*. Z. Zellforsch. **47**, 114—126 (1957).

Duncan, Donald: An electron microscope study of the neurohypophysis of a bird, Gallus domesticus. Anat. Rec. **125**, 457—471 (1956).

Fujita, H.: Electron microscopic observation on the neurosecretory granules in the pituitary posterior lobe of dog. Arch. hist. jap. **12**, 165—172 (1957).

Green, J. D., and V. L. van Breemen: Electron microscopy of the pituitary and observations on neurosecretion. Amer. J. Anat. **97**, 177—228 (1955).

Palay, S. L.: An electron microscope study of the neurohypophysis in normal, hydrated and dehydrated rats. Anat. Rec. **121**, 384 (Abstract No. 247) (1955).

— The fine structure of the neurohypophysis. Progr. Neurobiol. II. Ultrastructure and Cellular Chem. of Neural Tissue 31—49 (1957).

Schiebler, Th. H.: Cytochemische und elektronenmikroskopische Untersuchungen an granulären Fraktionen der Neurohypophyse des Rindes. Z. Zellforsch. **36**, 563—576 (1952).

Department of Anatomy, University of Uppsala, Sweden

Neurosecretory and Related Phenomena in the Hypothalamus and Pituitary of Man

By

P. O. LUNDBERG

With 5 Figures

When viewing the literature about neurosecretion in human hypothalami it soon becomes obvious that there are discrepancies between the observations of different authors. The early investigations of GAUPP and SCHARRER (1935) and others describe large amounts of "colloids" in the nucleus supraopticus (n. so.) and paraventricularis (n. pv.). In the more recent studies of HILD (1952) and PALAY (1953) only very few neurosecretory cells were found in the two nuclei. In chrome hematoxyline phloxine (GOMORI) preparations the intense ink-blue staining of the posterior pituitary is striking in contrast to the scanty reaction in the two magnocellular nuclei. Most of the research about human hypothalamus concerns these nuclei, but in a few papers (f. ex. RANSTRÖM, 1947), where other parts of the tuber cinereum are investigated, findings of granular intracellular products are mentioned.

Having had the opportunity to obtain a considerable number of human brains, most of them fixed within a few hours after death, the present author selected about 60 adult cases, 3 children, and 15 embryos without gross pathological involvement of the brain. The hypothalami and pituitaries were fixed mostly in Bouin or alcohol, paraffin imbedded, and after sectioning stained with chrome hematoxyline phloxine (GOMORI), paraldehyde fuchsin (GOMORI), alcian blue, gallocyanine, periodic acid Schiff, performic acid Schiff, Scharlach R, and some silver stains. Acid-fastness, reducing capacity, and ferric iron content were tested with the common methods. Unstained sections were studied in phase microscopy, darkfield illumination, and ultraviolet light.

Irrespective of the stain used, one of the most striking features in the human n. so. and n. pv. is the rich vacuolization. In chrome hematoxyline phloxine stained preparations of Bouin fixed materials most of the vacuoles appear empty or weakly acidophile, but some of them contain a clump stained blue-black. In a few cells of each 10 μ section, there are more or less homogeneous masses of distinctly blue-black droplets or filamentous formations. These droplets are more copious in the neurites.

In van Gieson preparations on the other hand, especially if the tissue is alcohol fixed, most vacuoles are filled with light-red, hyaline masses. In a few cells darker formations appear, sometimes within a vacuole. Also with many other methods it is possible to separate two different types of substances; one staining red in van Gieson preparations and the more sparsely distributed material staining blue with Gomori's chrome hematoxyline. It seems probable that the first one is what Divry (1934), Gaupp and Scharrer (1935), Peters (1936), and others called neurosecretory "colloid", and that the second one is what Hild (1952), Palay (1953), and Bargmann (1954) designated as neurosecretory material. These may well be two different substances. The van Gieson "colloid" sometimes extends a little in the neurites, but it is never found outside the regions of the n. so. and n. pv. The substance staining blue with chrome hematoxyline, however, behaves in human beings just as previously has been described in dogs and rats. There are neurites in the tractus hypophyseus loaded with blue staining material, formed like strings of pearls, and Herring bodies, sometimes with their characteristic acidophile centre and sometimes with a distinct acidophile membrane surrounding this centre. The Herring bodies may be as big as 100 μ in length; histochemical studies of their centre do not support the opinion that they are degenerating nerve cells. Among the capillary loops in the infundibulum and posterior pituitary neurites containing granules staining ink-blue with chrome hematoxyline are especially frequent.

This same material also stains with paraldehyde fuchsin and alcian blue after the same oxidation procedure as in the chrome hematoxyline method according to Gomori (permanganate-sulphuric acid), but it is not stained by Scharlach R and it is PAS negative. However, the cells of the n. so. and n. pv. do not remain entirely unstained after the last two procedures. Two kinds of intensely coloured granules appear. The first are about 1—2 μ in size and collected in large masses in some of the smaller cells and neurites of the n. pv. The second are very minute grains diffusely scattered over the whole cell and sometimes in the proximal part of the neurite both in the n. so. and n. pv. These two kinds of PAS positive granules stain brilliantly with paraldehyde fuchsin even without oxidation. After a slight modification of the chrome hematoxyline method they also stain with this method. Thus, we have three morphologically and histochemically different types of substances which stain blue with Gomori's chrome hematoxyline (table 1). For the sake of simplicity these are in the following designated as type one (the PAS-negative material), type two (the PAS positive big granules), and type three (the PAS positive minute granules), respectively.

When investigating the tuber cinereum the following was found: In the nuclei tuberis laterales the cells are filled with uniform granules of the second type, extending far into the neurites. In some of the cells in the nucleus infundibularis there are from 1—4 μ big, often solitary, droplets with the staining properties of the second type. They appear in both the neurites and dendrites. In the nucleus mamillo-infundibularis collections of such granules are seen near the nucleus. Granules of the third type are, however, only within the pericarya of the n. so. and n. pv.

In the whole posterior pituitary granules with the morphology and the staining properties of the second type occur in worm-shaped formations, sometimes several hundred microns long. Near the capillary loops in the median eminence and in the pituicyte nests of the infundibular process the granules are very numerous and appear in bulb-shaped collections. They are often seen in the pituicytes, too. As an estimation, about half the amount of substances in the pars neuralis which stain blue with chrome hematoxyline are of the second type.

The morphological similarities between the phenomena interpreted as neurosecretory by previous authors and the above described granules are thus very conspicous. It is, however, not possible without physiological methods to prove that the granules of type two and three represent signs of neurosecretion.

To make any conclusions about the histochemistry of the granules of the second and third type is difficult in view of the risk of autolytic changes. It is clear,

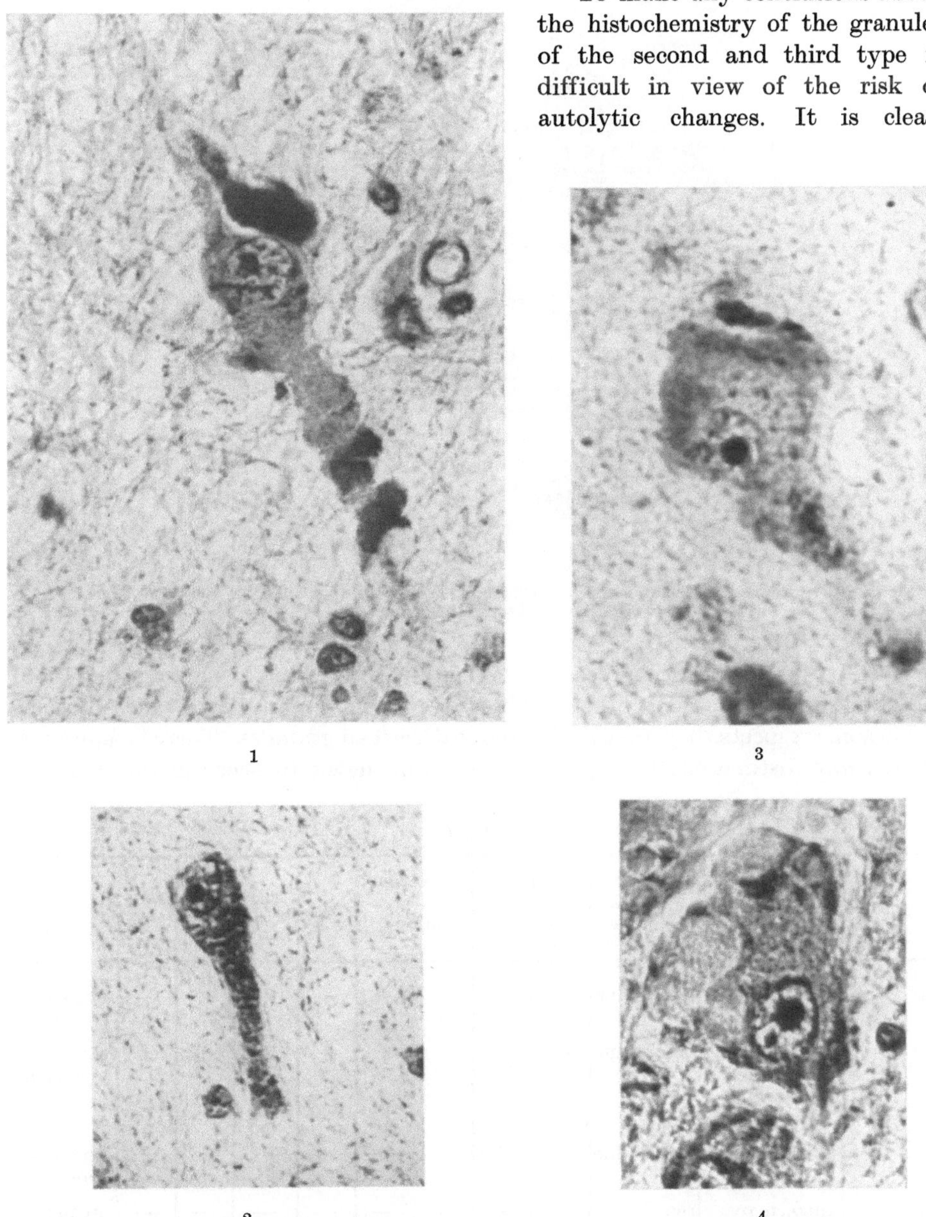

Fig. 1—3. Chrome hematoxyline phloxine (GOMORI). Bouin fixed. Fig. 1. Nucleus supraopticus. Black-blue clumps in the perikaryon with the staining properties of type one. 660 ×   Fig. 2. Nucleus infundibularis. Black-blue granules of the second type in the perikaryon and the neurite. 800 ×   Fig. 3. Nucleus supraopticus. Black-blue granules of the third type scattered over the perikaryon and at the neurite pole. 1000 ×
Fig. 4. Nucleus paraventricularis. Vacuoles with an acidophile content. Bouin. Azocarmine light green SF. 900 ×

however, that they are PAS positive and contain lipids. Granules with one of these qualities have earlier been noted in human hypothalamus by Gagel (1928), Poppi (1930), and Clara (1953). Poppi interpreted his findings as evidence of neurosecretion, and Clara his as lipofuscins. The histochemistry of central

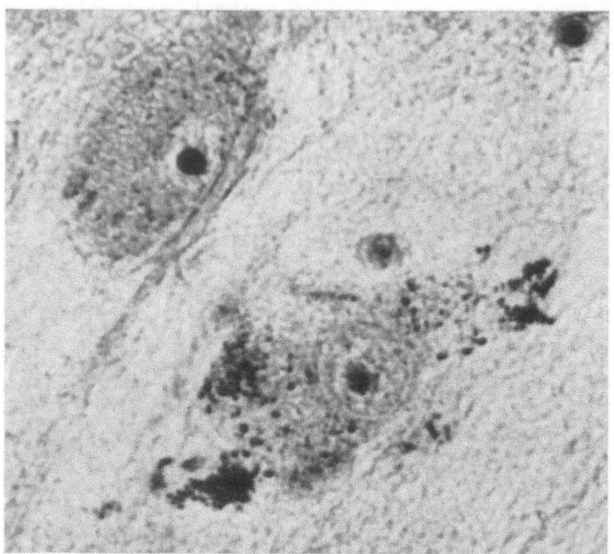

Fig. 5. Nucleus mamillo-infundibularis. Azocarmine-red granules in the pericaryon and in the processes. Bouin. Azocarmine. 900 ×

nervous lipofuscins has been recently studied by Dixon and Herbertsson (1950) and Sulkin (1953) among others. There seem to be many types of lipofuscins and in some respects they are like the above described granules. There is, however, one definite distinction: the lipofuscins are said never to occur in the neurites.

Table 1

Types	Presence in	Chrome hema- toxyline phloxine (Gomori)	Paraldehyde- fuchsin		Alcian blue		PAS	Schar- lach-R	Acid fast	Red. cap.	After alcohol fixation
			non ox.	ox.	non ox.	ox.					
one	n. so., n. pv.	black-blue	—	+	—	+	—	—	—	—	no reaction
two	n. inf., n.mam.inf., n.tub.lat. (n. pv.)	black-blue	+	+	(+)	+	+	+	+	+	slight reaction
three	n. so.	black-blue	+	+	—	—	+	+	+	—	no reaction
v. Gieson „colloid"	n.so., n.pv.	red	—	—	—	—	—	—	—	—	strong reaction
azocar- mine gra- nules	n.mam.inf.	red	—	—	—	—	—	—	—	—	same as after Bouin

The granules of the second type have probably nothing to do with the pituitary pigments, which are very easy to determine in darkfield illumination and do not contain any lipids.

In many of the cells of the nucleus mamillo-infundibularis one notes in chrome hematoxyline phloxine preparations hyaline droplets of different size staining red with phloxine. They are more distinctly coloured by azocarmine and in most respects quite different from the granules of the second type, which often occur in the same cell. The azocarmine granules also appear in the processes of the nerve cells, but it has not been possible to decide how far they extend. No such granules are found in the posterior pituitary.

Lastly, I will briefly mention the intranuclear "vacuoles" in the cells of the nucleus infundibularis. They have previously been described in Homo by ZIESCHE (1943) and HILD (1952) as "Kernkugeln". When one compares cells sectioned at different planes, one sees clearly that these "vacuoles" are cytoplasmic invaginations. These cells also show other irregularities in their nuclear membrane, and the cavities are more basophile than the rest of the cytoplasm. According to HYDÉN (1943) this may be interpreted as a sign of increased metabolism which perhaps has something to do with a possible neurosecretory function of the cells.

For the adult brains the findings, above described, are regular but they vary in quantity. No difference in relation to age or sex could be established.

Literature

BARGMANN, W.: Das Zwischenhirn-Hypophysensystem. Berlin-Göttingen-Heidelberg: Springer-Verlag 1954.
CLARA, M.: Psychiat. Neurol. med. Psychol. 5, 108—120 (1953).
DIVRY, P.: J. belge Neurol. Psychiat. 34, 649—658 (1934).
DIXON, K. C., and B. M. HERBERTSON: J. Path. Bact. 62, 335—339 (1950).
GAGEL, O.: Z. Anat. 87, 558—584 (1928).
GAUPP, R., und E. SCHARRER: Z. ges. Neurol. Psychiat. 153, 327—355 (1935).
HILD, W.: Z. Zellforsch. 37, 301—316 (1952).
HYDÉN, H.: Z. mikr.-anat. Forsch. 54, 96—130 (1943).
PALAY, S. L.: Amer. J. Anat. 93, 107—141 (1953).
PETERS, G.: Z. ges. Neurol. Psychiat. 154, 331—344 (1936).
POPPI, U.: Riv. Pat. nerv. ment. 36, 397—416 (1930).
RANSTRÖM, S.: Acta path. microbiol. scand. 70 (1947) Suppl.
SULKIN, M. N.: J. Geront. 8, 435—445 (1953).
ZIESCHE, K. T.: Z. Zellforsch. 33, 143—150 (1943).

From the Plymouth Laboratory of the Marine Biological
Association of the United Kingdom

Neurosecretory Transport in the Pituitary Stalk of Lophius piscatorius

By

D. B. CARLISLE

With 2 Figures

The pituitary stalk of the angler or goose fish, *Lophius piscatorius*, is notable for its length which may exceed 3 cm in a large fish. It is only about 50 μ thick and is accompanied by a hypophyseal portal vein. It is thus eminently suited for visual and electrical observations on the functioning of the pituitary stalk.

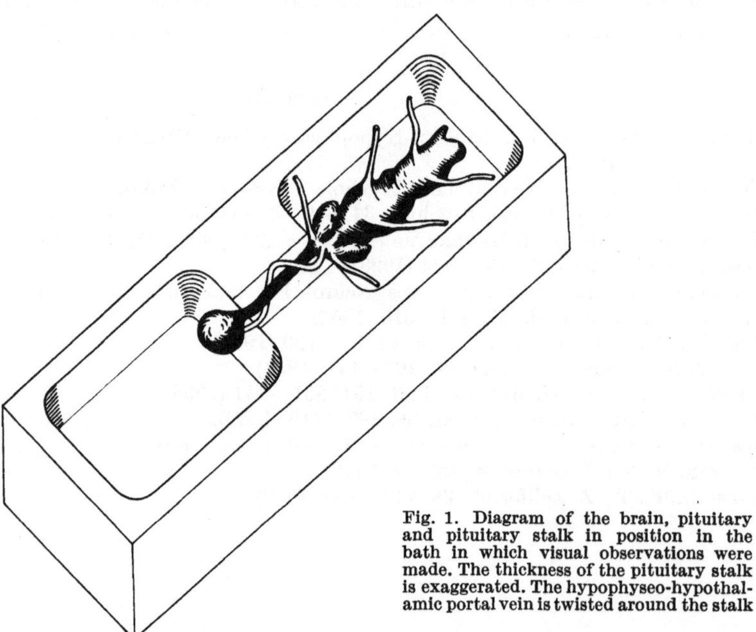

Fig. 1. Diagram of the brain, pituitary and pituitary stalk in position in the bath in which visual observations were made. The thickness of the pituitary stalk is exaggerated. The hypophyseo-hypothalamic portal vein is twisted around the stalk

Dr. DAVID POTTER informs me that 95% of the fibres which go to make up the stalk can be shown to contain neurosecretory material. For about three minutes after the removal of the brain, pituitary stalk and pituitary body from the animal the tissues remain translucent, thereafter they become progressively more opaque, a common symptom of moribundity in animal tissues. All visual observations were made during the first period of about three minutes. Electrical observations were perforce rather delayed since electrodes could not be applied accurately within this time, but some observations were made with the floor of the skull removed and the brain and pituitary body *in situ*.

With the normal light microscope intra-axonal objects could be observed migrating down a proportion of the axons, in most preparations. Some of these could be interpreted as mitochondria, but others, rather larger and of mulberry appearance, appeared to be conglomerations of neurosecretory material. They were quite unlike anything which I have observed in ordinary nerve fibres. These objects moved towards the pituitary at a rate of about 100—200 μ per minute. The movement ceased two or three minutes after removing the preparation from the body. The medulla of each fibre was of course birefringent, but the axon of a fibre in which no movement was taking place was nonbirefringent. The major axis of polarization of the medullary material was perpendicular to the axis of the axon, as would be expected. When axonal material is flowing the molecules tend to become orientated along the axon, thus producing a birefringence with the major axis of polarization along the axis of the axon. These two axes of polarization are thus perpendicular to one another and can therefore be distinguished as different colours with the use of a first order red gypsum slip in the polarization microscope. Under these conditions stationary axoplasm, streaming axoplasm and medullary material are distinguished as different colours, and the existence of streaming within the axons can be demonstrated.

In the film which was shown with the demonstration both moving "mulberries" and polarization effects with the three colours were shown as a direct record of neurosecretory movement within the pituitary stalk.

Electrical observations were made with the cathode ray oscilloscope. Both spontaneous activity and action potentials in response to stimulation of the stalk were recorded. The axons of the pituitary stalk of this species are thus capable both of neurosecretory transport intra-axonally and of the transmission of nervous impulses. It is not, however, clear whether both activities can go on in the same axon. These observations confirm the earlier findings of POTTER and LOEWENSTEIN (1955).

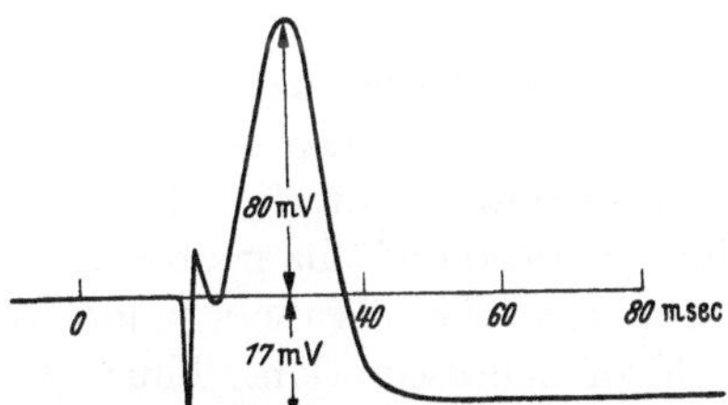

Fig. 2. An action potential of the pituitary stalk in response to a stimulus. The first small spike is the stimulus artifact, the main curve is the action potential. A tracing from a cathode ray oscilloscope record

Literature

POTTER, D. D., and W. R. LOEWENSTEIN: Electrical activity of neurosecretory cells. Amer. J. Physiol. **183**, 652 (1955).

Department of Morbid Anatomy, Charing Cross Hospital Medical School, London, England

The Application of Newer Histochemical and Isotope Techniques for the Localisation of Protein-bound Cystine or Cysteine to the Study of Hypothalamic Neurosecretion in Normal and Pathological Conditions

By

J. C. SLOPER

With 3 Figures

It is probable that the elaboration of the posterior pituitary principles is closely related to the secretion and storage of a hypothalamo-neurohypophysial neurosecretory material. It is suggested that histochemical techniques for the demonstration of this neurosecretory material should fulfill certain criteria which stem from the advances made by BARGMANN (1954) and his colleagues in the field of neurosecretion. Thus such histochemical techniques should be at least as selective as the Gomori chrome-alum-haematoxylin (CAH) staining method. Further the substances thus demonstrated should behave like material staining with CAH, both in the hypophysectomised animal, and in animals exposed to osmotic stress. The only histochemical techniques which satisfy these criteria demonstrate substances rich in protein-bound cystine or cysteine. Because of their selectivity and known histochemical basis they have a number of applications, in particular in comparative morphology and pathology. Their success has recently led us [ARNOTT and SLOPER (1957)] to attempt to study the dynamics of neurosecretion with the aid of radioactive (S^{35}) labelled cysteine.

Methods

The presence of protein-bound cystine and cysteine in neurosecretory material was first shown in 1954 by BARRNETT and SELIGMANN. Independent observations led later in the same year to similar conclusions [SLOPER (1954)], but more recent work has suggested that two of the techniques originally used, the alkaline tetrazolium of PEARSE, and the thioglycollate-dihydroxydinaphthyldisulphide technique of BARRNETT and SELIGMANN are not as selective as the CAH method, although BARRNETT (1954) was able to show depletion and accumulation of histochemically demonstrable neurosecretory material under the appropriate experimental conditions. On the other hand, the thioglycollate ferric-ferricyanide and performic acid Alcian blue (PFAB) techniques for protein bound cystine or cysteine fully satisfy the criteria mentioned above [SLOPER (1955); ADAMS and SLOPER (1956)]. Recently we have found that it is advisable to perform the

performic acid oxidation by dropping the acid on the dry section; also HUMBER-
STONE (personal communication) has obtained better staining by using a Crystal
violet-Dextrin-Resorcin fuchsin mixture instead of Alcian blue. 0.1 gm of the

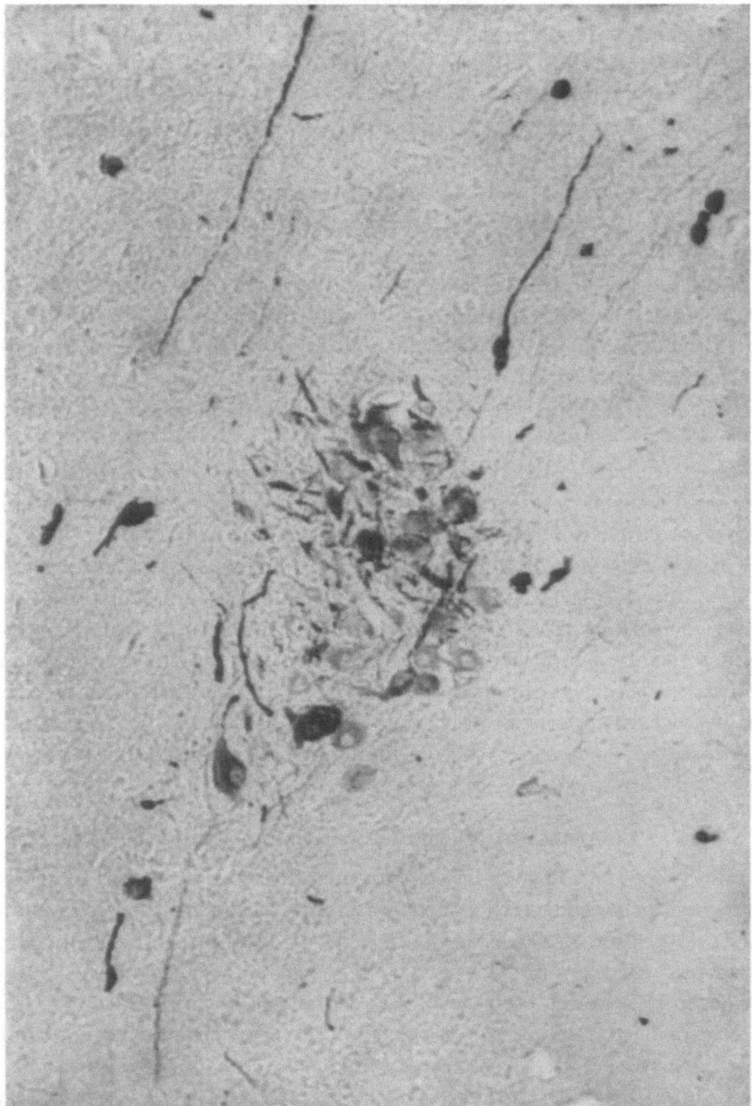

Fig. 1. Hypothalamus of dog. Neurosecretory cells and beaded fibres in region between nucleus paraventricularis
and nucleus supraopticus. Note selective staining of cystine-rich neurosecretory material. This reaction is given
equally intensely by material in the posterior lobe of the pituitary. Performic acid — Crystal violet, dextrin,
resorcin-fuchsin technique. 180 ×

dry precipitate of this stain is dissolved in 100 ml of 70 per cent. alcohol containing
6 ml of concentrated hydrochloric acid, and oxidised sections are stained for
three hours (Fig. 1). These techniques are used after formol-fixation, the effects

of which on sulfhydryl groups are discussed by Gomori (1955). Neurosecretory material can be demonstrated in alcohol-extracted unfixed tissues, provided such tissues are subsequently fixed in formalin before further processing.

General Applications

These histochemical techniques are more selective than the CAH and aldehyde fuchsin (AF) methods. Since cystine is a widespread constituent of the proteins of the brain, it is likely that the selectivity of these methods reflects their relative insensitivity, and thus the high local concentration of the amino-acid. In this respect material thus demonstrated shares a property of the protein with posterior pituitary activity isolated by Van Dyke and his coworkers (1942), which contains over five times the amount of cystine present in extracts of brain [Block and Bollings (1945)].

It is tempting to equate the two artefacts, the histological produced by treatment of the tissue with formalin, heat, water and various lipid solvents; and the biological, that is the preparation derived for bioassay from tissues subjected to the procedures used for the extraction of proteins. It is suggested that the cystine-rich protein demonstrated histochemically may be closely akin to the protein hormone, in whatever state the latter exists in the body. This view is the opposite of that held by Hild and Zetler (1953), who claimed that CAH neurosecretory material was a bearer substance, which, because of its solubility in lipid solvents, could not represent the hormone.

The selectivity of these histochemical techniques suggests their use in photometry. We have attempted this (Hansen, Einarson, Sloper, unpublished) by photographing serial sections from the paraventricular nuclei of normal rats, and of rats administered hypertonic saline. These nuclear regions were mounted at almost the same level in one paraffin block. This method largely overcomes variations in section-thickness and staining intensity, but it is too uncertain to be recommended, because of the difficulty of mounting the nuclear regions of test and control animal at the same level.

Comparative Morphology of Neurosecretion

The analogy between invertebrate and vertebrate neurosecretion [Hanström (1941)] was strengthened by the successful application of the CAH method to invertebrates [B. Scharrer (1951)]. Neurosecretory material in the pars inter-cerebralis-corpus cardiacum system of the cockroach, *Leucophaea maderae*, is equally selectively stained by the PFAB technique [Sloper (1957)]. For this reason, acetic acid extracts were made from retrocerebral tissue containing the corpora cardiaca dissected from 22 cockroaches *(Periplaneta americana)*. These extracts exhibited neither antidiuretic nor oxytocic activity when tested by Dr. Bisset in the rat by methods involving the intravenous injections of the extracts, and the use of the isolated rat uterus. These findings are not in accordance with those made by Stutinsky (1953) in the fly, but corroborate the unpublished observations of Hild and of Vogt [Scharrer (1955)]. Nevertheless, in spite of the apparent absence of a common biological activity in extracts made from the corpus cardiacum and posterior pituitary, it is possible that there are closely similar neurosecretory proteins in vertebrates and invertebrates alike.

Pathological Applications

The CAH and AF techniques, if used without counterstains, stain in different degree Nissl substance, nuclear chromatin, material in the background, and "lipofuscins", the latter term being used in a broad sense to include substances giving a wide variety of histochemical reactions [PEARSE (1953)]. For this reason, and because the chemical basis of these techniques is obscure, it is advisable to use histochemical techniques in the study of the pathology of the hypothalamo-hypophysial system. This applies particularly to the study of the accumulations of CAH material which develop proximal to lesions in the pituitary stalk. These accumulations contain material rich in cystine. However, we have also observed in them acidic substances, possibly acid mucopolysaccharides, that is, substances which might well be demonstrated by the basic dyes used in the CAH and AF techniques [SLOPER and ADAMS (1956)].

Selective histochemical techniques are also of value in the study of the development of retrograde degeneration in injured neurosecretory cells. Recent observations on hypophysectomised subjects suggest that the ability of the cell to form neurosecretory material is lost between 17 and 42 days after operation. It is of interest that some hypophysectomised human subjects do not develop overt diabetes insipidus, in spite of the administration of cortisone. This we have correlated with the presence of a large number of surviving cells containing cystine-rich material in the caudal part of the paraventricular nuclei, cells whose axones presumably end in the median eminence. In these patients, unlike the rats studied by STUTINSKY (1951) and by BILLENSTIEN and LEVEQUE (1953), there was no persistent accumulation of neurosecretory material in the surviving neurohypophysis. It is possible that in these rats, a greater proportion of neurosecretory cells survived than in the human subjects we studied, in whom hypophysectomy was performed for the relief of malignant disease.

(S^{35}) Labelled Cysteine and the Dynamics of Neurosecretion

ARNOTT and I have attempted to study the dynamics of neurosecretion with the aid of (S^{35}) labelled cysteine. We postulated that this amino-acid would be selectively taken up by the hypothalamo-hypophysial neurosecretory system. On this premise, it was likely to be concentrated, first in the supraoptic and paraventricular nuclei and later, depending upon the rate of flow of neurosecretory material in the axone, in the infundibular process of the posterior pituitary. Accordingly (S^{35}) DL cysteine was prepared by thioglycollate reduction from (S^{35}) DL cystine, and made up in a solution at p_H 6.7 containing in each 0.1 ml the equivalent of 0.19 mgm cystine, with a specific activity of 37.7 microcuries. This amount, injected intraperitoneally into rats of between 50 and 65 gm, was not selectively taken up by any part of the brain. Intracisternal injections were made in a second and similar series of rats, which, like those in the first series, were sacrificed by decapitation 5 minutes, 30 minutes, 5 hours (two rats), 17 hours, 24 hours and 96 hours after injection. Radioautographs revealed a selective uptake of (S^{35}) by the supraoptic nuclei, (Figs. 2 and 3), and to a lesser extent by the paraventricular nuclei, as compared with the adjacent hypothalamus. This was most marked in the animals sacrificed 30 minutes after injection.

However, only in the animal sacrificed 17 hours after injection was the uptake in the infundibular process markedly greater than in the adjacent hypothalamus.

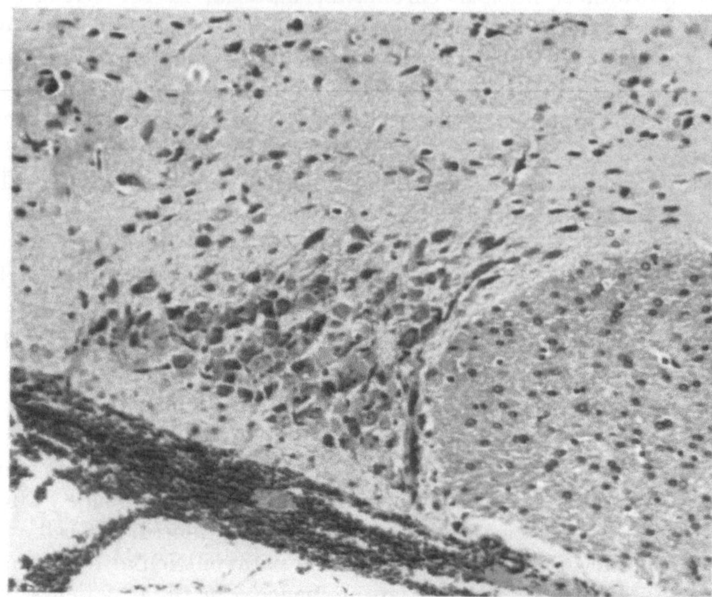

Fig. 2. Sagittal section through supraoptic nucleus of rat, sacrified 30 min. after intracisternal injection of (S³⁵) DL Cysteine, to show general morphology. Haematoxylin and eosin. 280 ×

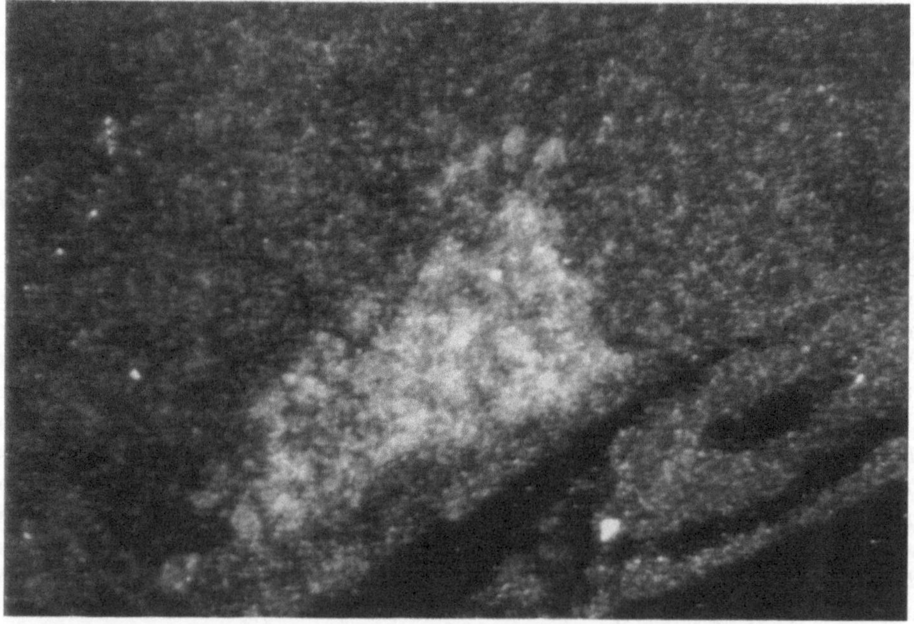

Fig. 3. Sagittal section through supraoptic nucleus of same rat as in Fig. 2 (Strip film autoradiograph). Note the accumulation of silver granules in emulsion overlying supraoptic nuclear region. Granules photographed under dark ground illumination. 280 ×

In a third series of rats the peak uptake by the infundibular process as compared with adjacent structures (hypothalamus, pars distalis) occurred 14 hours after injection, an observation corroborated by measurements made on 8 rats with a windowless Geiger counter on weighed dried samples of temporal cortex, cortex from the supraoptic region, and anterior pituitary and posterior pituitary. These observations we propose to amplify in further series. Meanwhile, in view of GAITONDE and RICHTER's (1955, 1956) work with (S^{35}) labelled methionine it is possible that a high proportion of labelled cysteine in our experiments was incorporated in protein. The late peak uptake of (S^{35}) by the infundibular process could therefore reflect the arrival of cystine-rich neurosecretory material in the posterior pituitary. On these premises the rate of flow of neurosecretory material is of the order of several millimetres a day. It should, however, be stressed that we do not know whether the radioactive sulphur was contained in protein, nor again can it be assumed that any of this sulphur reached the posterior lobe of the pituitary via its stalk. Nevertheless, it is probable that we have here a new and useful means of studying neurohypophysial function.

References

ADAMS, C. W. M., and J. C. SLOPER: J. Endocr. **13**, 221 (1956).

ARNOTT, D. J., and J. C. SLOPER: In preparation.

BARGMANN, W.: Das Zwischenhirn-Hypophysensystem. Berlin: Springer 1954.

BARRNETT, R. J.: Endocrinology **55**, 484 (1954).

— and A. M. SELIGMANN: J. nat. Cancer Inst. **14**, 769.

BILLENSTIEN, D. C., and T. F. LEVEQUE: Endocrinology **56**, 704 (1955).

BLOCK, R. J., and D. BOLLING: The amino-acid composition of proteins and food. Springfield, Ill. 1945.

DYKE, H. B. VAN, B. F. CHOW, R. C. GREEP and A. ROTHEN: J. Pharmacol. **74**, 109 (1942).

GAITONDE, M. K., and D. RICHTER: Biochem. J. **59**, 690 (1955).

— — Proc. roy. Soc. B **145**, 83 (1956).

GOMORI, G.: Quart. J. micr. Sci. **97**, 1 (1955).

HANSTRÖM, B.: Acta Univ. Lund., N. F. Avd. 2, **37**, No. 4, 1 (1941).

HILD, W., and G. ZETLER: Z. ges. exp. Med. **120**, 236 (1953).

LENDRUM, A. C.: In Recent Advances in Clinical Pathology. 2nd ed. p. 533, 1951.

PEARSE, A. G. E.: In Histochemistry, p. 364. London 1953.

SCHARRER, B.: Anat. Rec. **111**, 554 (1951).

— In The Hormones. vol. III p. 57. (PINCUS, G., and K. V. THIMANN, eds.) New York: Academic Press Inc. 1955.

SCHIEBLER, T. H.: Acta anat. (Basel) **13**, 233 (1951).

— Z. Zellforsch. **36**, 563 (1952).

SLOPER, J. C.: J. Anat. (Lond.) **88**, 576 (1954).

— J. Anat. (Lond.) **89**, 301 (1955).

— Nature (Lond.) **179**, 148 (1957).

— and C. W. M. ADAMS: J. Path. Bact. **72**, 307 (1956).

STUTINSKY, F.: C. R. Soc. Biol. (Paris) **145**, 367 (1951).

— Bull. Soc. Zool. France **78**, 202 (1953).

Zoologisches Institut der Universität, Helsinki, Finnland

Neurosekretion und Stress

Von

P. Suomalainen

Das von Selye dargestellte sog. allgemeine Adaptationssyndrom hat in der physiologischen und medizinischen Literatur immer hervorragendere Bedeutung erhalten. Experimentelle und klinische Beobachtungen haben gezeigt, daß der Organismus sich an Mikrobeninfektionen, Belastungen und Gewebsschäden in zweierlei Weise anpassen kann. Es können gewisse spezifische Adaptationsreaktionen vor sich gehen. Ein Beispiel hierfür sind die von vielen Krankheitserregern hervorgerufenen serologischen Gegenreaktionen. Der Organismus kann sich aber auch in unspezifischer Weise an den Zustand anpassen, der entsteht, wenn er belastet oder geschädigt wird, wenn er in Kälte oder Hitze kommt, wenn er im Hungerzustand gehalten wird, wenn man ihn mit einer gewissen Krankheit infiziert, ihm bestimmte Chemikalien injiziert oder Traumen zufügt. Alle diese unspezifischen Faktoren sind Stressoren, ihre Gesamtheit heißt Stress, und die Kombination der vom Stress hervorgerufenen unspezifischen Adaptationen ist das allgemeine Adaptationssyndrom ("general adaptation syndrome") von Selye. Nach Selye ist diese Reaktion keineswegs durch die Qualität der Stressoren bedingt, sondern durch die individuelle Reaktionsweise und den Abwehrmechanismus des Organismus.

Der Stoff, der den Säugetierkörper schnell in einen gewissen Bereitschafts- oder Alarmzustand versetzt, ist bekanntlich das Adrenalin, das sich plötzlich im Organismus ausbreitet und dessen allgemeine Funktionsfähigkeit steigert. Wenn der Stress weitergeht, reizt das Adrenalin die Adenohypophyse zur Sekretion von ACT-Hormon an, unter dessen Einwirkung die Nebennierenrinde anschwillt. Die Folge davon ist das allgemeine Adaptationssyndrom, von welchem verschiedene Phasen unterschieden werden. Die erste ist die sog. „Alarmreaktion", d. h. der Organismus geht zur Defensive über. Der Stressor erzeugt zuerst eine Schockphase, auf welche aber bald die Gegenschockphase folgt, wobei die ganze Widerstandsfähigkeit des Individuums mobilisiert wird. Sobald die Abwehrmaßnahmen des Organismus sich stabilisiert haben, folgt die Widerstandsphase der Selyeschen Reaktion. Die Hormonsekretion der Nebennierenrinde ist ständig größer als normal und der Organismus verteidigt sich erfolgreich. Wenn aber dieser Zustand lange andauert, so scheint die Abwehrenergie des Organismus aufgebraucht zu werden und es tritt die letzte Phase des Selyeschen allgemeinen Adaptationssyndroms ein, nämlich die Erschöpfungs- oder Kollapsphase, in welcher die Widerstandskraft des Organismus zusammenbricht.

Ich habe mit meinen Mitarbeitern schon längere Zeit die Physiologie des Winterschlafes untersucht. Mein Versuchstier ist der Igel *(Erinaceus europaeus* L.*)*.

Der charakteristischste Spezialzug in der Physiologie des Winterschlafes ist die Umstellung des Säugetieres von Homoiothermie zu Poikilothermie (vgl. z. B. Suomalainen und Suvanto). Der Winterschlaf ist daher ein natürlicher hypothermischer Zustand, aber auch ein lange andauernder Hungerzustand. Sowohl Kälte als auch Hunger rufen eine kräftige Alarmreaktion hervor. Unsere Untersuchungen über die Zahlenverhältnisse der Blutkörperchen und über die Histophysiologie der Nebennierenrinde haben gezeigt [Suomalainen (1954, 1956)], daß der Winterschlaf ein Zustand von schwerem Stress ist (Neutroleukocytose, Eosinopenie, Lymphopenie, Hypertrophie und aktivierte Tätigkeit der Nebennierenrinde). Das allgemeine Adaptationssyndrom spielt in der Physiologie des Winterschlafes eine ausschlaggebende Rolle.

Tabelle 1. *Die relative Größe der Kerne des Nucleus supraopticus beim Igel in verschiedenen Jahreszeiten*

Aktiv			Im Winterschlaf		
Im Juni	2,97		Im November-Dezember	3,80	
	2,60			3,85	
	3,50	3,02		4,26	
Im Juli	3,46			4,42	4,08
	3,52		Im Januar	4,80	
	2,93	3,30		5,34	
Im August	3,58			4,28	4,81
	3,63		Im Februar	4,62	
	3,68	3,63		5,35	
Im September-Oktob.	3,44			4,53	4,83
	3,82		Im März	5,05	
	3,63			4,75	
	4,35			5,40	5,07
	3,73	3,79	Im April	4,61	
				4,30	
				4,30	4,40
			Aktiv		
			Im Mai	3,41	
				3,50	
				2,89	3,27

Das Tier nimmt im Winterschlaf kein Wasser zu sich. Da jedoch der Stoffwechsel dann hauptsächlich auf der Konsumierung von Fetten beruht, entsteht im Körper des Winterschläfers von selbst verhältnismäßig reichlich Wasser. Die Hämatokritprozente des Blutes scheinen unseren Bestimmungen gemäß während des Winterschlafes wenig zu steigen (Suomalainen und Nyholm). Aber aus allem zu schließen, muß der Igel im Winterschlaf Wasser sparen. Aus diesem Grunde haben wir in letzter Zeit die Neurosekretion des Hypothalamus untersucht (Suomalainen und Nyholm).

Da die objektive quantitative Schätzung der Neurosekretionsgranula schwierig ist, haben wir die Größe der Zellkerne des Nucleus supraopticus als Maß für die Aktivität der Zellen benutzt; das funktionelle Kernödem von Benninghoff. Mit dem Zeichenapparat wurden von jedem Tier 100 Kerne des Nucleus supraopticus mit 1500facher Vergrößerung gezeichnet. Die relative Größe der Kerne wurde dann mit dem Planimeter bestimmt. In der Tab. 1 sehen wir die Mittelwerte. Wie aus der Tabelle ersichtlich ist, sind die Kerne im Juni am kleinsten.

Im Juli-August und in der prälethargischen Periode im September-Oktober werden die Kerne fortdauernd größer. Die Kerne der winterschlafenden Igel sind immer größer als die der aktiven Tiere. Am größten sind sie im März und werden während des Winterschlafes in der postlethargischen Periode im April wieder kleiner.

Die Resultate von unseren Untersuchungen über die Größe der Zellkerne und das histophysiologische Bild des Hypothalamus-Hypophysen-Systems (vgl. Suomalainen und Nyholm) kann ich folgenderweise zusammenfassen.

1. Die Neurosekretion ist im Sommer offenbar ziemlich schwach.

2. In der prälethargischen Periode im Herbst ist die neurosekretorische Tätigkeit aktiver, aber das Sekret wird in der Neurohypophyse gespeichert.

3. Die Neurosekretion ist während des Winterschlafes intensiv. Nur im Hochwinter kann man in der Neurohypophyse gespeichertes Sekret sehen.

Die Beziehungen zwischen Wasserstoffwechsel und Neurosekretion sind schon längere Zeit bekannt [vgl. z. B. Bargmann (1954) u. a.]. Die winterschlafenden Tiere müssen Wasser sparen und so ist das Bedürfnis nach dem antidiuretischen Prinzip im Winterschlaf offenbar größer als bei Sommertieren. Das erhöhte Bedürfnis nach der antidiuretischen Substanz in dehydrierten Tieren geht parallel mit der Entleerung der Neurohypophyse von dieser Substanz und mit der Vergrößerung der Zellkerne des Hypothalamus.

Diesmal interessieren uns die Beziehungen zwischen Neurosekretion und Stress. Wie ich schon in einem anderen Zusammenhang beschrieben habe [Suomalainen (1954)], ist der Igel schon in der prälethargischen Periode im September-Oktober unter dem Einfluß von schwachem Stress. Die Nebennierenrinde ist aktiviert und die Neurosekretion ist gleichzeitig intensiver geworden, was eine schwache Alarmreaktion bedeutet. 2 oder 3 Wochen vor dem Beginn des Winterschlafes sind das allgemeine Adaptationssyndrom und gleichzeitig die neurosekretorische Aktivität noch stärker. Der beginnende Winterschlaf im Frühwinter verursacht keine größeren Veränderungen im allgemeinen Adaptationssyndrom; die Widerstandsphase scheint fortzudauern. Der starke Frost im Hochwinter aktiviert die Nebennierenrinde. Zu gleicher Zeit ist auch die Neurosekretion aktiver. Die physiologische Widerstandsfähigkeit des Igels erreicht ihr Maximum im Spätwinter. Die Neurosekretion ist aber auch in dieser Zeit am intensivsten. Die Korrelation zwischen Neurosekretion und dem allgemeinen Adaptationssyndrom ist hier also sehr deutlich.

Wie Bargmann schon im Jahre 1955 betont hat, stellt die Neurohypophyse nur ein Speicherorgan dar, das durch Stress verschiedener Natur in morphologisch und pharmakologisch faßbarer Weise zur Entleerung gebracht werden kann. Das neurosekretorische System antwortet also ähnlich der Nebennierenrinde mit ihrer sog. Alarmreaktion auch auf unspezifische Reize.

Meine eigenen Untersuchungen haben eine ganz deutliche Korrelation zwischen der Neurosekretion des Winterschlafes und des durch die Hypothermie verursachten Stress ergeben. Diese setzt jedoch eine physiologische Brücke zwischen der Neurosekretion und der Adenohypophyse voraus. Stein und Mirsky sowie E. Scharrer haben kürzlich dieses interessante und wichtige Verhältnis behandelt. Scharrer findet es als ziemlich erwiesen, daß das Neurosekret auch denjenigen Faktor, ein gewisses Peptid, enthält, der die Sekretion von ACTH regelt und dadurch eine Brücke von den vegetativen Zentren des Hypothalamus zur Adenohypophyse und damit zu den Nebennieren bildet. Die Zeit erlaubt es mir nicht, hier die Untersuchungen zu referieren, die dieser Auffassung zugrundeliegen. Ich erwähne lediglich beispielsweise solche Forscher wie MARTINI und MORPURGO, GUILLEMIN und HEARN, SAFFRAN, SCHALLY und BENFEY, MIRSKY und STEIN, und verweise auf die oben mitgeteilten Zusammenfassungen von STEIN und MIRSKY sowie von E. SCHARRER.

Literatur

BARGMANN, W.: Das Zwischenhirn-Hypophysensystem. Berlin-Göttingen-Heidelberg 1954.
— Die funktionelle Morphologie der Hormonbildungsstätten. Klin. Wschr. **1955**, 322—328.
BENNINGHOFF, A.: Kernschwellungen und Kernschrumpfungen.Anat.-Kongr. Bonn 1949.
SCHARRER, E.: Neurosecretion. In: Fifth Annual Report on Stress. H. SELYE and G. HEUSER, Eds. Montreal; Acta Inc. 1956, p. 185—192.
SELYE, H.: The stress concept in 1955. In: Fifth Annual Report on Stress. H. SELYE and G. HEUSER. Eds. Montreal: Acta Inc. 1956, p. 25—103.
STEIN, M., and I. A. MIRSKY: The relation between anterior and posterior hypophysis and the hypothalamus in response to stress. In: Hypothalamic-Hypophysial Interrelationships. W. S. FIELDS, R. GUILLEMIN and C. A. CARTON, Eds. Springfield, 1956, p. 58—73.
SUOMALAINEN, P.: Further investigations on the physiology of hibernation. Proc. Finn. Acad. Sci. **1953**, 131—144 (1954).
— Hibernation, the natural hypothermia of mammals. Triangle **2**, 227—233 (1956).
— and P. NYHOLM: Neurosecretion in the hibernating hedgehog. In: BERTIL HANSTRÖM. Zoological Papers in Honour of his sixty-fifth Birthday November 20th, 1956, p. 269—277. Lund 1956.
— and I. SUVANTO: Studies on the physiology of hibernating hedgehog. I. The body temperature. Ann. Acad. Sci. fenn. A **4**, 20, 1—20 (1953).

Aus dem Max-Planck-Institut für Hirnforschung, Neuroanatomische Abteilung in Gießen
(Prof. SPATZ) und dem Neurologischen Institut (Edinger-Institut) der Universität Frankfurt
am Main (Prof. KRÜCKE)

Über Begleiterscheinungen der Neurosekretion im Silberbild

Von

J. CHRIST, FR. ENGELHARDT und R. DIEPEN

Mit 7 Abbildungen

Einleitung

Die derzeitigen Vorstellungen der Neurosekretionslehre sind im wesentlichen durch die Beobachtungen von SCHARRER (1928—1933 u. sp.) an den *Zellen* des Nucleus praeopticus, bzw. supraopticus und paraventricularis bei niederen und höheren Wirbeltieren bestimmt. Die späteren Untersuchungen von BARGMANN (ab 1949) mittels der Gomori-Methode[1] haben insofern zu einer entscheidenden Erweiterung und Differenzierung der ursprünglichen Befunde geführt, als sie den Ausgangspunkt experimenteller Untersuchungen abgaben. Die Ansichten über die Produktion, Ableitung und Abgabe des Sekretes wurden somit hauptsächlich auf Grund *cytologischer* Beobachtungen bei Anwendung histologischer Färbemethoden entwickelt, wobei der Schwerpunkt bei den *sekretorischen* Phänomenen *am Zelleib* der Neurone der großzelligen Kerne — des Nucleus supraopticus und des Nucleus paraventricularis — im Hypothalamus lag; die Neuriten dieser Zellen wurden — etwa analog den Verhältnissen bei exokrinen Drüsen — lediglich als eine Art Ausführungsgänge angesehen. Die Feinstrukturen, wie sie vor allem im Infundibulum und im Hinterlappen vorkommen, blieben dabei unbeachtet und ebenso wurde der Neuronencharakter der sekretorisch tätigen Ganglienzellen nicht berücksichtigt. Die morphologische Erforschung eines so ungewöhnlichen Phänomens, wie wir es in der Produktion von färberisch darstellbaren Sekretsubstanzen und offenbar auch von aktiven Wirkstoffen [HILD und ZETLER (1951)] durch zentrale Neurone vor uns haben, verlangt unseres Erachtens jedoch gerade die Berücksichtigung der Feinstrukturen, die nicht nur Aufschluß über den histologischen Aufbau dieser Neurone geben, sondern auch über ihre Reaktionsform. Zur Darstellung solcher besonders differenzierter histologischer Phänomene bedarf es aber neben der Gomorifärbung der Anwendung geeigneter Silberimprägnationsmethoden.

In dieser Mitteilung werden einige Befunde am neurosekretorischen System in Silberpräparaten[2] und ihre Beziehungen zu den Phänomenen im Gomori-

---

[1] Hier und im folgenden ist damit immer die von BARGMANN zuerst bei der Untersuchung der neurosekretorischen Phänomene im Hypophysenzwischenhirnsystem verwandte Chromalaunhämatoxylin-Phloxin-Methode von GOMORI gemeint.

[2] Bei unseren Untersuchungen haben wir in der Hauptsache die Silbermethoden von BODIAN und PALMGREN angewandt.

Präparat besprochen, welche unsere Kenntnisse über die den Sekretionsvorgang begleitenden gestaltlichen Veränderungen an den supraoptico-hypophysären Neuronen ergänzen sollen und unter Umständen geeignet sein könnten, die Grundlagen der Vorstellungen über den Ablauf des sekretorischen Geschehens zu erweitern. Wir stützen uns dabei auf vergleichende Untersuchungen bei verschiedenen Säugetieren [cf. DIEPEN und ENGELHARDT (1958)], beschränken uns in der vorliegenden Arbeit aber auf·die Verhältnisse beim Menschen und beim Hund als kontrastierende Beispiele bezüglich der Gesamtmenge und der Verteilung des Neurosekretes innerhalb des Systems.

Da es uns darauf ankam, etwaige Zusammenhänge zwischen den Phänomenen des Silberbildes und dem Sekretionsprozeß festzustellen, waren Paralleluntersuchungen an Gomori-Präparaten erforderlich. Um darüber hinaus Aufschluß über die Konstanz von Entsprechungen zwischen Silberbild und Gomori-Präparat zu erhalten, wurden die Befunde bei mehreren Säugetieren [DIEPEN (1955), DIEPEN et al. (1958), GOSLAR (1952)] kontrolliert. Dabei war zu berücksichtigen, daß in der Säugetierreihe zwischen den einzelnen Arten Unterschiede bezüglich der Gesamtmenge, sowie bezüglich der Verteilung der neurosekretorischen Substanz auf die verschiedenen Abschnitte des Systems bestehen. Beim Menschen und beim Hund sind diese Unterschiede besonders deutlich ausgeprägt, so daß sie als ,,extreme Typen" der genannten Verhältnisse für vergleichende Untersuchungen am besten geeignet schienen: Beim *Menschen* findet sich innerhalb des gesamten Systems im ganzen sehr viel weniger Gomori-Substanz als beim Hund, wobei diese zugleich *fast ausschließlich auf den Hinterlappen* beschränkt ist; das Kerngebiet und die Tuberstrecke sind nach unseren Erfahrungen beim Menschen so gut wie frei von Gomori-Substanz und im Infundibulum begegnet man im allgemeinen nur vereinzelten Herringkörpern und feinen Perlschnurfasern. Beim *Hund* dagegen enthält *das ganze System*, außerdem von den Ursprungszellen und dem Hinterlappen, auch die Zwischenstrecke im Tuber cinereum und im Infundibulum, besonders große Sekretmengen. *Die Masse* des Sekretes findet sich allerdings auch hier *im Hinterlappen*, der beim Normaltier stets mit Gomori-blauen Granula und Tropfen angefüllt ist.

Befunde

Die bekanntesten Phänomene im Silberbild der Neurohypophyse beim Menschen und bei den Säugetieren sind die eigenartigen *Endkolben* neurosekretorischer Fasern, sowie losgelöste, freiliegende *Kugeln.* In beiden Fällen ist vielfach eine fibrilläre Struktur nachweisbar. Sie sind bereits von einer Reihe von Autoren beschrieben worden [TELLO (1912), BUCY (1932), TROSSARELLI (1935), HAIR (1938), ROMEIS (1940), HANSTRÖM (1946 u. sp.), HAGEN (1950, 1952), CHRIST (1951), BRETTSCHNEIDER (1954) u. a.], jedoch gehen deren Ansichten über die Natur und Bedeutung dieser Gebilde auseinander. Entgegen der seinerzeit von HAIR und von ROMEIS vertretenen Auffassung, daß es sich bei den ersteren um besondere, nicht mit anderen färberisch darstellbaren Gebilde identische nervöse Endapparate[1] handeln soll, dürfte heute feststehen, daß die Kolben und Kugeln — zumindest zum Teil — den sog. *Herringkörpern* entsprechen (BUCY, TROSSARELLI, HANSTRÖM, HAGEN, CHRIST, BRETTSCHNEIDER). Auf Grund der Tatsache, daß die Herringkörper sich mit GOMORIs Hämatoxylin blauschwarz anfärben, kann außerdem mit Sicherheit angenommen werden, daß die Endkolben und Kugeln Beziehungen zum Sekretionsvorgang besitzen. Nach BARGMANN (1949) stellen die Herringkörper neurosekrethaltige Verdickungen der marklosen Axone dar.

---

[1] Wobei offenbar an Terminalgebilde analog motorischen und sensiblen Endorganen usw. gedacht ist.

Mit diesen Feststellungen ist allerdings nach unserer Auffassung die eigentliche Natur dieser Gebilde noch nicht eindeutig bestimmt. Tello, der sie wegen ihrer Ähnlichkeit mit entsprechenden Bildungen an pathologisch-veränderten Nervenfasern als „bolas de degeneración" bezeichnete, nahm an, daß sie tatsächlich Anzeichen eines degenerativen Zerfalls der neurohypophysären Nervenfasern darstellen. Andere Autoren sahen in den Endkolben für die sekretorischen Fasern spezifische Endorgane der sekretorischen Fasern (Hanström, Brettschneider), die sich unter Umständen vom Axon lösen und in die Kugeln umwandeln können (Hanström). Eine Mittelstellung nimmt etwa Hagen (1949, 1950, 1952, 1955) ein, die einerseits Beziehungen zur neurosekretorischen Funktion für möglich hält, andererseits „pathologische Veränderungen" oder „Reizerscheinungen" an den Nervenfasern in Erwägung zieht. In ihren späteren Veröffentlichungen scheint Hagen unter der Vorstellung einer „physiologischen Degeneration" mehr zu der zuerst genannten Auffassung zu neigen.

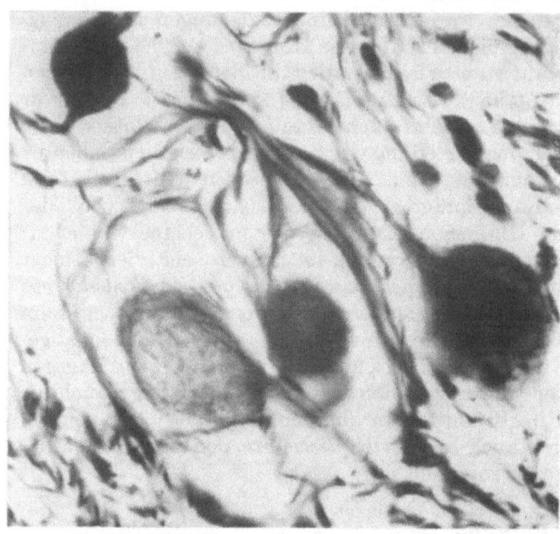

Abb. 1. Nervöse Endkolben aus dem Hinterlappen des Hundes. Eine fibrilläre Struktur ist lediglich bei dem linken Kolben zu erkennen, während bei den übrigen, nahezu homogen schwarz imprägnierten Kolben nur stellenweise eine undeutliche Struktur sichtbar ist. — Fix. Bouin, Paraffin 15 μ, Silberimprägnation nach Palmgren. Vergr. 750mal

Die genauere Untersuchung ergibt, daß es sich bei den Endkolben tatsächlich um Phänomene handelt, wie man sie neben anderen unten angeführten Veränderungen regelmäßig nach traumatischer Schädigung oder experimenteller Durchschneidung peripherer und zentraler Nervenfasern am Stumpf des proximalen, noch im Zusammenhang mit dem Zelleib befindlichen Axonabschnittes beobachtet. Die Endkolben (s. Abb. 1) — die ihrerseits aus umschriebenen, spindelförmigen Axonauftreibungen hervorgehen — können sich vom Axonstumpf ablösen und dann längere Zeit im Gewebe liegen bleiben. Ihnen entsprechen die auch in der Neurohypophyse anzutreffenden isolierten Kugeln (Abb. 2).

Der eine von uns [Christ (1951)] hat in einer früheren Mitteilung bereits seine Ansicht über die Natur dieser Bildungen und über ihre Beziehungen zum Sekretionsvorgang angedeutet und dabei die Möglichkeit eines unter physiologischen Bedingungen vor sich gehenden Zerfalls von Nervenfasern im Rahmen des Sekretionsvorganges angenommen.

Die Vorstellung, daß die Sekretproduktion mit einem Zerfall und Untergang von Neurobzw. Axoplasma einhergeht, ist im Hinblick auf den Sekretionsmodus echter Drüsenzellen durchaus nicht ungewöhnlich; man denke z. B. an Talgdrüsen, deren Sekret mit einiger Berechtigung als Produkt einer fettigen Degeneration der Drüsenzellen aufgefaßt werden könnte. Der Zerfall von Zellsubstanz bzw. ganzer Zellen wird — und zwar unter normalen Bedingungen — aber auch bei endokrinen Drüsen (Nebenniere, Ovar, Zwischenzellen des

Hodens) beobachtet[1]. Diese Interpretation trifft jedoch im Zentralnervensystem wegen der im allgemeinen noch festgehaltenen Vorstellung von einer — unter physiologischen Bedingungen — morphologischen Konstanz des Neurons auf gewisse Schwierigkeiten. Wie unsere weiteren Befunde nahelegen, läßt sich diese Ansicht aber — wenigstens bezüglich der sekretorisch tätigen Neurone — kaum noch aufrecht erhalten (auch bei einem partiellen Zerfall des Neurons, evtl. mit anschließender Regeneration, kann von einer Konstanz des Neurons u. E. nicht mehr die Rede sein).

Weitere Beobachtungen ähnlicher Natur ergeben ganz eindeutig eine Stütze für die vorhin geäußerte Auffassung. Außer den nervösen Endkolben und den Kugeln finden sich in der Neurohypophyse im Silberbild weitere, ebenfalls aus der Neuropathologie und durch experimentelle Untersuchungen bekannte Phänomene, die mit Sicherheit als *Reaktions- und Zerfallsphänomene* der Nervenfasern aufzufassen sind.

Beim Menschen wie beim Hund kommen im Verlauf der supraoptico-hypophysären Nervenfasern oft *Verdickungen*, *Schwellungen*, sowie umschriebene, spindelige *Auftreibungen* (meist leichten Grades, Abb. 3), vor, und zwar hauptsächlich innerhalb der Infundibulumstrecke (weniger häufig in der Tuberstrecke[2] selbst und im Hinterlappen). Diese Erscheinungen fassen wir z. T. als vermutlich noch reversible reaktive Veränderungen auf. Es kann sich dabei um Veränderungen leichteren Grades handeln, die im extremen Fall zur Bildung der Endkolben und Kugeln (Herringkörper) führen. Sie gleichen den nach experimenteller Durchschneidung oder traumatischer Durchtrennung in früheren Stadien, sowohl proximal von der Durchschneidungsstelle wie auch am distalen Axonfragment, beobachteten Veränderungen. In der Neurohypophyse wurden derartige Erscheinungen bisher wohl deswegen kaum beschrieben, weil sie — insbesondere bei unzulänglicher bzw. unvollständiger Imprägnation — innerhalb der dichten Faserbündel des Tractus supraoptico-hypophyseus leicht zu übersehen sind (s. Abb. 3)[3].

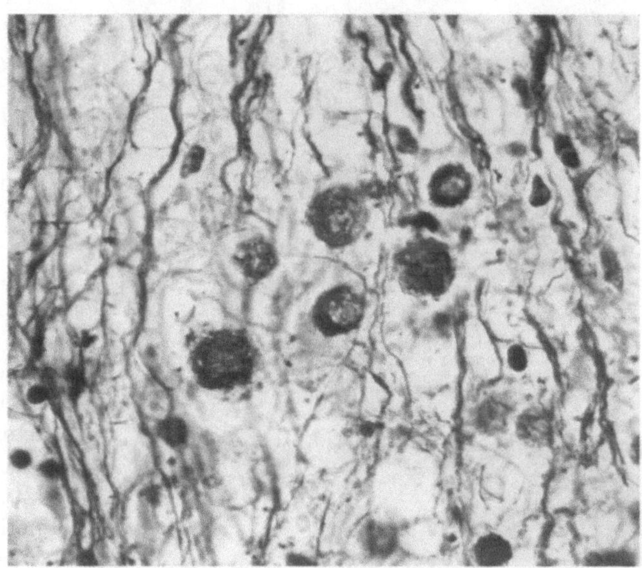

Abb. 2. Eine Gruppe freiliegender Kugeln beim Menschen im distalen Abschnitt des Infundibulum, unmittelbar beim Übergang in den Hinterlappen. Die Fasern des an dieser Stelle deutlich gelichteten Tractus supraoptico-hypophyseus sind teilweise verdickt, „verbacken" und auffällig gewellt. Fix. Bodian 3, Paraffin 15 μ, Silberimprägnation nach BODIAN. Vergr. 650mal

---

[1] cf. WATZKA: Handbuch der allgemeinen Pathologie 2, 1 (1955).

[2] Bezüglich der Terminologie siehe bei DIEPEN, ENGELHARDT und SMITH-AGREDA (1954).

[3] Die photographische Wiedergabe hat zwar den Nachteil, daß gerade bei starker Vergrößerung stellenweise erheblich Unschärfen auftreten, jedoch haben wir sie der Zeichnung vorgezogen, um subjektive Momente, die bei der zeichnerischen Darstellung kaum vermeidbar sind, auszuschließen.

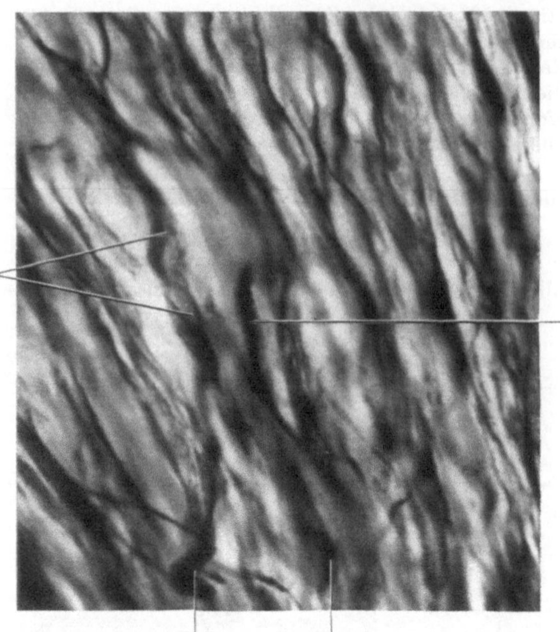

Abb. 3. Ausschnitt aus dem Tractus supraoptico-hypophyseus des Hundes beim Übergang von der Tuberstrecke in das Infundibulum. Unregelmäßige Verdickungen und „Quellungen" (×). Fix. Bouin, Paraffin 15 μ, Silberimprägnation nach Palmgren. Vergr. 1100mal

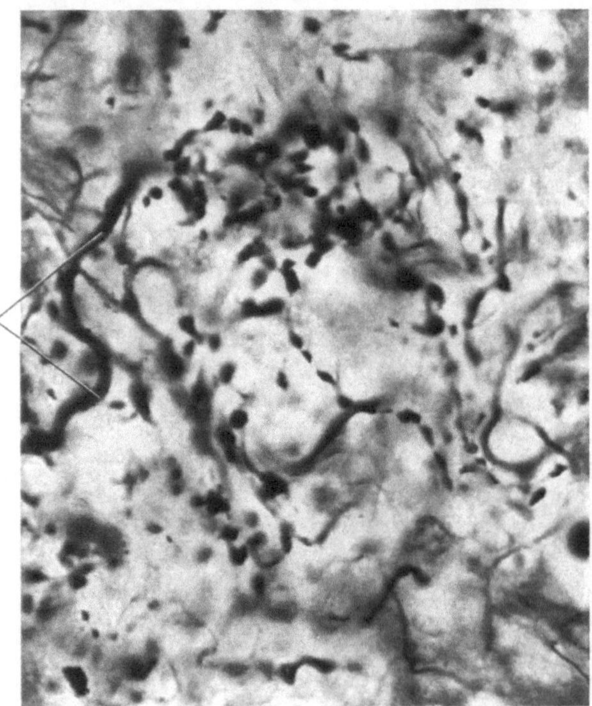

Abb. 4. Perlschnurartig veränderte Nervenfaserendigungen und grob-granulärer Zerfall in einer perivasculären „Verdichtungszone" des Hinterlappens beim Hund. Bei × ein stark verdicktes und „wurmförmig" gekrümmtes Faserfragment. Fix. Bouin, Paraffin 15 μ, Silberimprägnation nach Palmgren. Vergr. 1100mal

Neuen Erscheinungen begegneten wir im Silberbild im Hinterlappen, und zwar in den perivasculären Verdichtungszonen und — beim Hund — in der an den Zwischenlappen angrenzenden Randzone, also in den Gebieten der Endaufsplitterungen der supraoptico-hypophysären Nervenfasern. In diesen Gebieten fanden wir *perlschnurartig veränderte* Endabschnitte (s. Abb. 4), sowie ungleichmäßig, z. T. besonders intensiv, z. T. nur blaß imprägnierte, ferner *verdickte* und *unregelmäßig gekrümmte Axonfragmente* (s. Abb. 4). Es handelt sich hierbei um die gleichen charakteristischen Bilder, wie sie nach schwereren mechanischen oder andersartigen Schädigungen von Nervenfasern häufig beschrieben worden sind [Cajal (1913, 1928), Spatz (1921), Herzog (1952)[1]]. Die perlschnurartig veränderten Fasern und Faserabschnitte dürften wohl z. T. mit den von Knoche (1952, 1953), u. a. im Hinterlappen beschriebenen ‚Nodulusfasern' identisch sein. Häufig jedoch fehlen die zarten Verbindungsstücke zwischen den Verdickungen, die dann mehr rundliche grob-granuläre Gestalt angenommen haben, und schließlich finden sich

---

[1] Siehe auch bei Seitelberger (1956).

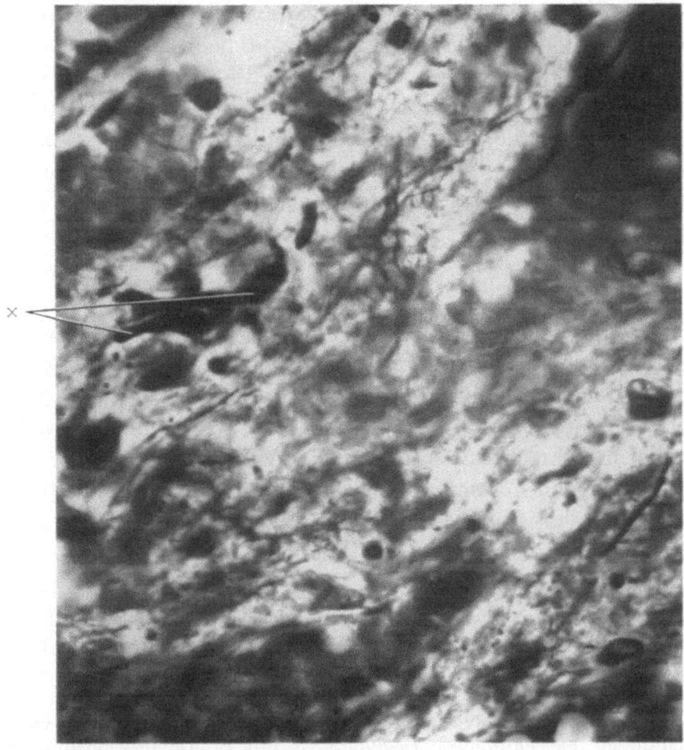

Abb. 5. Faserzerfall in der Übergangszone zum Hinterlappen beim Menschen. Bei × unförmig verdickte und bizarr deformierte Nervenfaserfragmente. Ferner zeigt die Abbildung noch weitere weniger stark veränderte Axonfragmente und Anzeichen eines feingranulären Zerfalls. Charakteristischerweise finden sich die Veränderungen hauptsächlich in Gefäßnähe. Fix. Bodian 3, Paraffin 15 μ, Silberimprägnation nach BODIAN. Vergr. 750mal

Gebiete, die das Aussehen eines granulären, unter Umständen staubförmigen Zerfalls besitzen, so daß der Eindruck eines Trümmerfeldes entsteht, in welchem

gelegentlich noch gröbere, unförmig verdickte, bizarr geformte Axonfragmente anzutreffen sind (Abb. 5).

Im Hinblick auf die in der Einleitung erwähnten im Gomori-Präparat beobachteten Unterschiede zwischen den Verhältnissen beim Menschen und denen beim Hund, ist die Tatsache von Interesse, daß im Silberpräparat die Zerfallserscheinungen im Hinterlappen beim

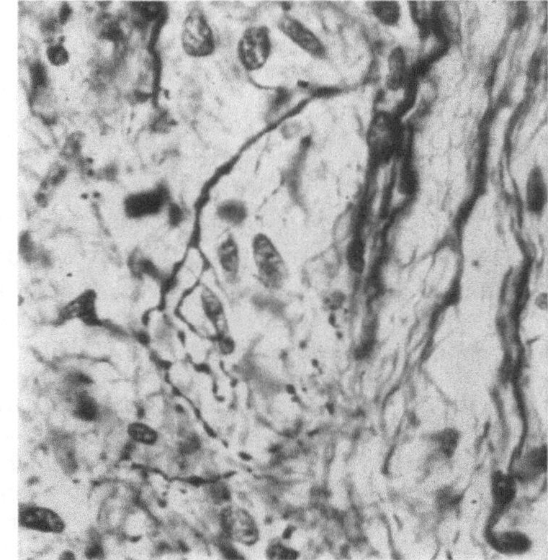

Abb. 6. Perlschnurartige Veränderung des sich dichotomisch aufsplitternden Endabschnittes einer neurosekretorischen Faser aus dem Hinterlappen des Hundes. Der Faserabschnitt proximal von der Teilungsstelle fällt bereits durch seine unregelmäßige Kontur auf. In der Umgebung sieht man freiliegende Zerfallsgranula. Fix. Bouin, Paraffin 15 μ, Silberimprägnation nach PALMGREN. Vergr. 600mal

3*

Menschen weniger zahlreich bzw. weniger ausgesprochen (und daher auch weniger leicht auffindbar) sind, als beim Hund. Ferner sind beim Menschen die Granula wesentlich feiner und es gelingt daher nur selten die Beziehungen von reihenförmig hintereinanderliegenden Körnchen zu noch intakten Faserabschnitten nachzuweisen. Beim Hund kann man dagegen häufig Fasern bis in ihre dichotomischen Verzweigungen verfolgen und dabei die distalwärts zunehmende Veränderung der terminalen Abschnitte bis zum Zerfall in immer kleiner werdende Granula beobachten (s. Abb. 6).

Diskussion

Angesichts dieser ungewöhnlichen Befunde liegt es nahe, zunächst an Artefakte zu denken. Diese Möglichkeit kann unseres Erachtens jedoch — vor allem im Hinblick auf die übrigen geschilderten Veränderungen in den weiter proximal gelegenen Abschnitten des Systems — mit Sicherheit ausgeschlossen werden. Wir halten es für völlig unwahrscheinlich, daß es auf Grund methodischer Mängel zur Ausbildung von Artefakten kommt, welche insgesamt die aus der Pathologie und vom Experiment her bekannten Reaktions- und Zerfallserscheinungen von Nervenfasern in solcher Vollständigkeit nachahmen.

Wie die Experimente von Cajal, Spatz u. a. gezeigt haben, treten z. B. nach experimenteller Durchschneidung peripherer und zentraler Nervenfasern — außer am Zelleib — immer auch ganz charakteristische Veränderungen am zentralen, noch mit dem Zelleib zusammenhängenden Axonabschnitt sowie am peripheren, isolierten Fragment auf, und zwar handelt es sich dabei — im proximalen Abschnitt — um Verdickungen, Auftreibungen, Bildung von Endkolben und Fibrillenkugeln. Bei dem peripheren vom Zelleib getrennten Fragment stehen die Erscheinungen der sekundären Degeneration mit Fragmentation und granulärem Zerfall, vor allem im Bereich der am weitesten distal gelegenen Abschnitte, im Vordergrund. Die Art und Intensität der Veränderungen hängt bekanntlich vom Ort der Kontinuitätsunterbrechung, d. h. deren Abstand vom Zelleib, ab. Ferner ist zu berücksichtigen, daß bei besonders feinen marklosen Axonen (wie wir sie in den terminalen Aufsplitterungen des Hinterlappens vor uns haben) auch ohne Kontinuitätsunterbrechung oder sonstige schwere mechanische Schädigung, auf Grund toxischer (chemischer) Einwirkungen ein primärer granulärer Zerfall eintreten kann. Auf die charakteristischen gestaltlichen Veränderungen am Zelleib, die vor allem bei Anwendung der Nissl-Methode zu erkennen sind, soll in diesem Zusammenhang nicht eigens eingegangen werden. Wir möchten lediglich nochmals auf die bekannte Ähnlichkeit der Ganglienzellen des Nucleus supraopticus und des Nucleus paraventricularis mit anderen durch Überbelastung aktivierten Ganglienzellen hinweisen.

Die Vorstellung, daß in der Neurohypophyse an den Nervenfasern unter physiologischen Bedingungen und im Rahmen eines physiologischen Vorganges Zerfallserscheinungen vorkommen, findet eine Stütze in den neueren Befunden einer hochgradigen Regenerationsfähigkeit derselben Nervenfasern bei Tractusdurchschneidung und nach Hypophysektomie [Gaupp und Spatz (1955), Billenstein und Leveque (1955), Jörgensen, Rosenkilde und Wingstrand (1956), Moll (1957), Engelhardt und Diepen (im Druck); Vortragsreferat in Endokrinologie 34, 349 (1957); Escolar (1958)].

In diesem Zusammenhang ist es wichtig, darauf hinzuweisen, daß sich nicht nur die zum Zerfall führende Reaktion morphologisch in der Form von Perlschnurfasern und Kugeln manifestiert, sondern auch der Vorgang, der im Zuge der Regeneration stattfindet. Genau wie bei anderen Neuronen spielen sich also an den supraoptico-hypophysären Neuronen, sowohl bei „regressiven", wie bei den reparativen Vorgängen die erwähnten charakteristischen Veränderungen ab, die wir als „Neuronale Reaktionsweise" verstehen und bezeichnen. Dabei ist allerdings ein grundsätzlicher Unterschied gegenüber anderen Neuronen zu beachten: Nur die supraoptico-hypophysären Neurone zeigen die Phänomene der neuronalen Reaktionsweise *auch* im Gomoribild. Wir fanden z. B. bei der Ratte drei Wochen nach Läsion der supraoptico-hypophysären Neurone im Gomoribild gewucherte (gomorigefärbte) Regenerate in Form von Perlschnurfasern und Endkolben (ENGELHARDT u. DIEPEN 1958).

Wir glauben ferner, daß gewisse Entsprechungen im Gomoribild, die auf enge Beziehungen zum Sekretionsvorgang hindeuten, ebenfalls gegen die Deutung unserer Befunde als Artefakte sprechen: Betrachten wir einmal die quantitativen Verhältnisse, so zeigt sich, daß die neuronalen Reaktionserscheinungen und Zerfallsphänomene beim Menschen insgesamt gegenüber dem Hund weniger zahlreich bzw. weniger intensiv sind. Dem entspricht die beim Menschen im Gomoripräparat deutlich geringere Gesamtmenge von Neurosekret innerhalb des ganzen Systems. Darüber hinaus findet sich auch in den einzelnen Abschnitten des Systems eine Parallelität bezüglich des Gehaltes an Gomorisubstanz einerseits und des Auftretens der Faserveränderungen im Silberbild andererseits. Am deutlichsten ist dies im Hinterlappen: Beim Vergleich aufeinander folgender Schnitte, von denen einer nach der Palmgren-Methode behandelt und der andere nach GOMORI gefärbt ist, ergibt sich, daß die dichtesten Ansammlungen von Neurosekret-Granula und -Tropfen gerade in den Regionen vorkommen, in welchen die Zerfallserscheinungen der Nervenfasern am stärksten ausgeprägt sind, d. h. in den perivasculären Verdichtungszonen sowie in der Randzone des Hinterlappens. Die Abb. 7a u. b läßt dies deutlich erkennen[1]; man sieht u. a., daß der Bereich der noch in Bündeln parallel verlaufenden Nervenfasern (die „Zwischenstreifen" von ROMEIS) kaum Gomorisubstanz aufweist, während das Gebiet der Endaufsplitterungen große Massen von Sekret enthält.

Wenn auch diese Entsprechungen zweifellos auf eine Beziehung zwischen den reaktiven bzw. den Zerfallserscheinungen der Nervenfasern einerseits und der Sekretbildung andererseits schließen lassen, so ist aber durchaus keine durchgängige Identität der im Silberpräparat dargestellten Phänomene mit den Gomori-positiven Strukturen anzunehmen. So finden sich beim Hund z. B. in der Tuberstrecke bei der Gomori-Färbung bekanntlich zahlreiche „Perlschnurfasern", während das Silberpräparat keine entsprechenden Phänomene bietet. Ebenso findet sich im Hinterlappen eine „Dissoziation" der Phänomene insofern, als die argentophilen Zerfallsgranula nicht mit den Gomori-Granula gleichgesetzt werden können. Bei der Beurteilung der Befunde kann man daher nicht über die Feststellung einer topographischen *Entsprechung* hinausgehen, die angesichts ihrer Konstanz jedoch genügend Anhalt bietet, die sekretorischen Vorgänge zu den Reaktions- und Zerfallserscheinungen in Beziehung zu setzen. Auf die Beziehungen zwischen den neuronalen Phänomenen im Silberbild und den Gomori-färbbaren Strukturen im einzelnen soll in einer weiteren Veröffentlichung von CHRIST (im Druck) ausführlich eingegangen werden.

Beim Vergleich des Silberpräparates mit dem Gomoripräparat ergibt sich somit beim Menschen wie beim Hund sowohl eine allgemeine quantitative Parallelität zwischen den neuronalen Veränderungen im Silberbild und den Gomori-färbbaren Phänomenen, als auch eine Parallelität bezüglich der quantitativen Verteilung beider Phänomene innerhalb des Systems: Die Orte intensiver und ausgedehnter Faserveränderungen sind zugleich die Orte größeren Sekretreichtums und umgekehrt.

---

[1] Auf eine farbige Abbildung, die diese Entsprechungen wesentlich deutlicher zeigt, wurde aus äußeren Gründen verzichtet.

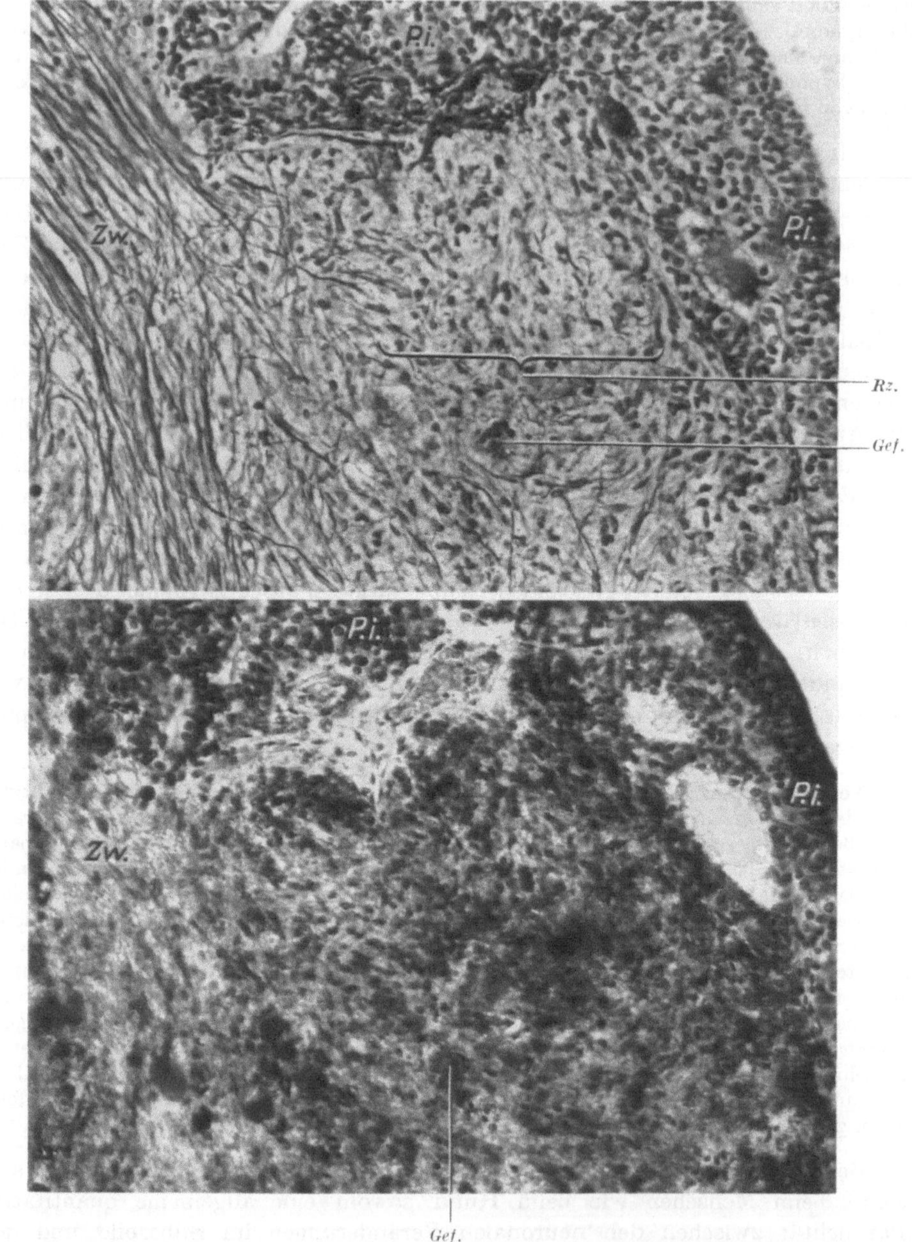

Abb. 7a u. b. a) Ausschnitt aus einem schrägen Horizontalschnitt durch den Hinterlappen des Hundes. Es ist ein Teilgebiet aus dem rechten vorderen Quadranten des Hinterlappens dargestellt. Links vom Hilus her in den Hinterlappen eintretende geschlossene Faserzüge („Zwischenstreifen"). Rechts daran anschließend die (periphere) an die Pars intermedia angrenzende Randzone des Hinterlappens, in der sich vorwiegend Endaufsplitterungen sowie die Zerfallsphänomene finden, die bei der schwachen Vergrößerung der Abbildung jedoch nicht zu erkennen sind. Fix. Bouin, Paraffin 15 μ, Silberimprägnation nach Palmgren. Vergr. 210mal. b) Ein benachbarter, nach Gomori mit Chromalaunhämatoxylin gefärbter Schnitt, der die im Text geschilderten Entsprechungen zwischen den Orten der Zerfallserscheinungen und den Gomori-färbbaren Phänomenen zeigt. Die korrespondierenden Stellen sind durch Hinweislinien gekennzeichnet. Deutlich ist die der Lokalisation der Zerfallserscheinungen entsprechende perivasculäre dichtere Lagerung der Gomori-Substanz. Gef. = Gefäß; Zw. = Zwischenstreifen; Rz. = Randzone; P. i. = Pars intermedia. Fix. Bouin, Paraffin 15 μ, Gomoris Chromalaunhämatoxylin- Phloxin- Färbung. Vergr. 210mal

Die mitgeteilten Befunde lassen mit Sicherheit auf einen Zusammenhang der im Silberbild festgestellten Faserveränderungen mit dem sekretorischen Geschehen schließen, wobei die Art des Zusammenhanges allerdings nicht ohne weiteres ersichtlich ist.

Wenn man bei dem (S. 32, unten) angeführten Beispiele bleibt, könnte man an eine Umwandlung des zerfallenden Neuro- bzw. Axoplasma in Sekret, d. h. Hormon denken, die Identität, oder zumindest eine enge Kopplung der färberisch darstellbaren Substanz mit den spezifischen Wirkstoffen vorausgesetzt. DIEPEN und ENGELHARDT (1958) [s. a. DIEPEN, ENGELHARDT und SMITH-AGREDA (1954)] haben im Hinblick auf die Feststellungen von HILD (1951), sowie von HILD und ZETLER (1951), wonach die Gomori-Substanz von den aktiven Wirkstoffen zu trennen ist, u. a. die Möglichkeit diskutiert, daß die färberisch darstellbare Substanz ein im Rahmen der Hormonbildung auftretendes „neuronales Phänomen" darstellt. Die Autoren begründen diese Ansicht mit dem charakteristischen „topistischen" Auftreten der Gomori-Substanz am Neuron, insofern, als in der Ontogenese wie auch innerhalb der Wirbeltierreihe die Gomori-Substanz in erster Linie in den Abschnitten festzustellen ist, in welchen sich bei geschädigten Nervenfasern im Silberbild die charakteristischen neuronalen Veränderungen finden: Das Verteilungsmuster der neurosekretorischen Substanz innerhalb des Systems in der Ontogenese sowie in der Wirbeltierreihe entspricht der zeitlichen Folge des Auftretens der Schädigungszeichen an pathologisch veränderten Nervenfasern, und zwar treten beide immer zuerst in den *distalen* Abschnitten des Neurons auf; *danach* zeigen sich die reaktiven Veränderungen am Zellkörper *und zuletzt* kommt es auch zu solchen an den dazwischen gelegenen Abschnitten des Neurons. Wir möchten die im Silberpräparat festzustellenden neuronalen Reaktions- und Zerfallserscheinungen zunächst *nur* als charakteristische neuronale Begleitphänomene der Neurosekretion ansehen und die Frage offen lassen, ob sie tatsächlich unmittelbare Schlüsse auf den Sekretionsmodus zulassen, d. h. ob sie das Wesen des Sekretionsvorganges (den Sekretionsmodus) der hormonbildenden Neurone bestimmende Veränderungen darstellen.

Auf Grund dieser Befunde sind wir zu der Ansicht gekommen, daß es sich bei dem färberisch darstellbaren Neurosekret nicht um eine, vom Zelleib distalwärts transportierte Substanz handelt. — Die Frage, ob die im Silberpräparat festgestellten Reaktions- und Zerfallserscheinungen tatsächlich unmittelbare, verallgemeinernde, Schlüsse auf den Sekretionsmodus dieser Neurone erlauben, d. h. ob sie das Wesen des Sekretionsprozesses (den Sekretionsmodus) darstellen, möchten wir noch offen lassen. CHRIST denkt daran, daß es sich um Phänomene handeln könnte, wie sie auch bei anderen endokrinen Drüsen unter physiologischen Bedingungen durch Überbeanspruchung funktionell weniger belastbarer sekretorischer Elemente vorkommen.

In der vorliegenden Mitteilung kam es uns in erster Linie darauf an, die bisher kaum berücksichtigten Phänomene an den Nervenfasern des Tractus supraopticohypophyseus *im Silberbild*, sowie ihren spezifisch neuronalen Charakter herauszustellen und dabei zugleich auf die eindeutigen Beziehungen dieser Veränderungen zu den Erscheinungen im Gomoripräparat (also zur Sekretbildung) hinzuweisen. Die Natur der bei Silberimprägnation an den supraoptico-hypophysären Nervenfasern in Erscheinung tretenden Phänomene kann mit deren Einordnung in das Schema der neuronalen Reaktions- und Desintegrationserscheinungen geklärt gelten. Eine endgültige Stellungnahme zur Frage ihrer Bedeutung für die Sekret- bzw. Hormonbildung sowie für die Vorstellungen über den Sekretionsmodus ist noch nicht möglich. Experimentelle Untersuchungen hierzu wurden durch ENGELHARDT und durch CHRIST bereits begonnen.

Die Arbeit wurde mit Unterstützung der Akademie der Wissenschaften und der Literatur, Mainz, durchgeführt.

Literatur

Bargmann, W.: Über die neurosekretorische Verknüpfung von Hypothalamus und Neuro-
hypophyse. Z. Zellforsch. **34**, 610—634 (1949).
— Das Zwischenhirn-Hypophysensystem. Berlin-Göttingen-Heidelberg: Springer 1954.
— and E. Scharrer: The site of origin of the hormones of the posterior pituitary. Amer.
Scientist **39**, 255—259 (1951).
Billenstien, D. C., and T. F. Leveque: The reorganization of the neurohypophyseal stalk
following hypophysectomy in the rat. Endocrinology **56**, 704—717 (1955).
Brettschneider, H.: Hypothalamus und Hypophyse des Pferdes. Morph. Jb. **96**, 265—384
(1954).
Bucy, P. C.: The hypophysis cerebri. In Penfield's Cytology and cellular Pathology of the
nervous system. Vol. 2, p. 705—742. New York: Hoeber 1932.
Cajal, S., Ramon y: Estudios sobre la degeneración y regeneración. Madrid: Hijos de Nicolas
Moya 1913.
— Degeneration and regeneration of the nervous system Vol. II. Oxford and London 1928.
Christ, J.: Zur Anatomie des Tuber cinereum beim erwachsenen Menschen. Dtsch. Z. Nerven-
heilk. **165**, 340—408 (1951).
Diepen, R.: Zur vergleichenden Anatomie des Hypophysen-Hypothalamus-Systems.
In: Die zentrale Steuerung der Sexualfunktion. I. Symposion dtsch. Ges. Endokrinol.
Hamburg 1953. S. 54—64. Berlin-Göttingen-Heidelberg: Springer 1955.
— u. Fr. Engelhardt: Neuronale Phänomene im Hypothalamus-Hinterlappensystem.
In: Pathophysiologia diencephalica. Symposion Mailand. S. 122—133. Wien: Springer 1958.
— — u. J. Christ: Neurosecretion as a neuronal process. Record I. internat. congress of
neurological sciences. Brüssel 1958 (im Druck).
— — u. V. Smith-Agreda: Über Ort und Art der Entstehung des Neurosekretes im supra-
optico-hypophysären System bei Hund und Katze. Anat. Anz. Erg. H. **101**, 276—288 (1954).
Engelhardt, Fr., und R. Diepen: Über Veränderungen am supraoptico-hypophysären
System nach Koagulationen in der Area medialis des Tuber cinereum. V. Symposion dtsch.
Ges. Endokrinol. Freiburg 1957. Berlin, Göttingen, Heidelberg: Springer 1958.
Escolar, J.: Vortrag 54. Anat. Kongreß (Freiburg), 1957.
Gaupp, V., u. H. Spatz: Hypophysenstieldurchtrennung und Geschlechtsreifung. Über
Regenerationserscheinungen an der suprasellären Hypophyse. Acta neuroveg. (Wien)
12, 285—328 (1955).
Goslar, H. G.: Vergleichende cytologische Untersuchungen zur Frage der Neurosekretion
im Hypothalamus. I. Acta neuroveg. (Wien) **4**, 381—408 (1952).
— Vergleichende cytologische Untersuchungen zur Frage der Neurosekretion im Hypo-
thalamus. II. Acta neuroveg. (Wien) **5**, 25—54 (1952).
Hagen, E.: Über die feinere Histologie einiger Abschnitte des Zwischenhirns und der Neuro-
hypophyse. II. Mitteilung. Acta anat. (Basel) **25**, 1—33 (1955).
Hair, G. W.: The nerve supply of the hypophysis of the cat. Anat. Rec. **71**, 141—160 (1938).
Hanström, B.: The hypophysis in a tiger (Felis tigris) and in an indian elefant (Elephas
maximus). Kgl. Fysiogr. Sällsk. Handl., Lund, N. F. **57**, 8 (1946).
— A comparative study of the hypophysis in the polar bear and some swedish carnivora.
Kgl. svensk. Vetensk. Akad. Handl., (Stockh.) Tredjeser. **24**, 7 (1947).
— The hypophysis in some south-african insectivora, hyracoidea, proboscidea, artiodactyla
and primates. Ark. Zool. (Stockh.) **4**, 187—294 (1952).
— The hypophysis in a wallaby, two tree-shrews, a marmoset, and an orang-utan. Ark. Zool.
(Stockh.) **6**, 97—154 (1953).
Herzog, E.: Histopathologie des vegetativen Nervensystems. Handbuch der speziellen
pathologischen Anatomie und Histologie (Henke-Lubarsch) XIII, 5. Berlin-Göttingen-
Heidelberg: Springer 1955.
Hild, W.: Vergleichende Untersuchungen über Neurosekretion im Zwischenhirn von Amphibien und Reptilien. Z. Anat. **115**, 459—579 (1951).
— u. G. Zetler: Über das Vorkommen der Hypophysenhinterlappenhormone im Zwischenhirn. Arch. exper. Path. Pharmak. **213**, 139—153 (1951).
— — Vergleichende Untersuchungen über das Vorkommen der Hypophysenhinterlappenhormone im Zwischenhirn einiger Säugetiere. Dtsch. Z. Nervenheilk. **167**, 205—214 (1952).

Jörgensen, C. B., P. Rosenskilde and K. G. Wingstrand: Regeneration of the neural lobe of the pituitary gland in the toad, Bufo bufo (L.). In B. Hanström, Zoological papers in honour of his 65th birthday etc., p. 184—195. Zool. Inst. Lund (publisher) 1956.

Knoche, H.: Neurohistologische Untersuchungen am Hypophysen-Zwischenhirnsystem des Hundes. Anat. Anz. Erg. H. 99, 93—95 (1952).

— Über das Vorkommen eigenartiger Nervenfasern (Nodulus-Fasern) in Hypophyse und Zwischenhirn von Hund und Mensch. Acta anat. (Basel) 18, 208—223 (1953).

Moll, J.: Regeneration of the supraoptico-hypophyseal and paraventriculo-hypophyseal tracts in the hypophysectomized rat. Z. Zellforsch. 46, 686—709 (1957).

Romeis, B.: Die Hypophyse. Handbuch der mikroskopischen Anatomie des Menschen (Möllendorff) Bd. VI, 3, S. 1—609. Berlin: Springer 1940.

Scharrer, E., u. B. Scharrer: Neurosekretion. Handbuch der mikroskopischen Anatomie des Menschen (Möllendorff-Bargmann) Bd. VI, 5, S. 953—1066. Berlin-Göttingen-Heidelberg: Springer-Verlag 1954.

Seitelberger, F.: Zur Morphologie und Histochemie der degenerativen Axonveränderungen im Zentralnervensystem. I. Congrès internat. des sciences neurologiques (III. congr. internat. neuropathologie). Les éditions Acta med. belg. (1957).

Spatz, H.: Über die Vorgänge nach experimenteller Rückenmarksdurchschneidung mit besonderer Berücksichtigung der Unterschiede der Reaktionsweise des reifen und des unreifen Gewebes nebst Beziehungen zur menschlichen Pathologie (Porencephalie und Syringomyelie). Nissl- u. Alzheimersche Arbeiten S. 49—364. Erg. Bd. Jena: Fischer 1921.

Tello, F.: Algunas observaciones sobre la histologia de la hipofisis humana. Trab. Lab. Invest. biol. Univ. Madrid 10, 145—184 (1912).

Trossarelli, A.: Eclaircissements sur l'histologie de la neurohypophyse. Bull. histol. appl. 12, 29—44 (1955).

Laboratoire d'Histologie de la Faculté de Médecine de Nancy, France

Les voies extra-hypothalamo-neurohypophysaires de la neurosécrétion diencéphalique dans la série des Vertébrés

Par

H. LEGAIT

Avec 8 Figures

L'existence de voies neurosécrétoires extra-hypothalamo-neurohypophysaires a été signalée dès le début de l'utilisation de la coloration de Gomori à l'hématoxyline chromique phloxine pour l'étude de l'hypothalamus. Les premières observations ont été faites chez les Reptiles. SCHARRER décrit dès 1951 chez *Thamnophis* une voie neurosécrétoire allant des noyaux paraventriculaires vers la commissure palliale postérieure et la base de la paraphyse. Incidemment HILD signale également des trajets neurosécrétoires vers la paraphyse et une région épendymaire richement vascularisée chez *Tropidonotus natrix* et *Vipera berus*. Plus récemment, la première description de SCHARRER a été étendue et vérifiée chez plusieurs autres Reptiles par ANANTHANARAYANAN (1955).

Chez le Poisson-Chat, STUTINSKY (1955) a également observé des chaînettes de grains neurosécrétés au niveau des ganglions habénulaires. Des observations comparables ont été effectuées également chez quelques Mammifères. BARGMANN (1954) décrit des trajets «Gomori-positifs» moniliformes dans l'épiphyse du Hérisson, ayant probablement la valeur de fibres neurosécrétoires. BARRY au laboratoire d'Histologie de Nancy (1954, 1955, 1956) a mis en évidence chez quelques Cheiroptères en état d'hibernation plusieurs voies extra-hypophysaires de la neurosécrétion diencéphalique.

Ces premières investigations semblaient par conséquent établir l'existence chez quelques Vertébrés de voies neurosécrétoires destinées à des centres nerveux autres que la neurohypophyse, situés à des distances importantes des noyaux hypothalamiques. La découverte fortuite d'un grand nombre de chaînettes de grains au niveau des ganglions de l'habenula de la Poule ainsi que le caractère fragmentaire des données recueillies par les auteurs précédents nous a incité à reprendre ces recherches chez les Oiseaux (1955), puis chez les Batraciens et les Reptiles (1956). Ces diverses investigations que nous résumerons au cours de cet exposé, ont pu être complétées récemment chez quelques Poissons et Mammifères; elles nous permettent d'affirmer que ce système de voies extra-hypothalamo-neurohypophysaires existe chez toutes les espèces étudiées et que le plan d'organisation de ce système semble comparable dans les différentes classes des Vertébrés.

Méthodes utilisées pour la mise en évidence des voies neurosécrétoires extra-hypophysaires

L'étude de ces voies extra-neurohypophysaires pose deux problèmes principaux: il s'agit en premier lieu de trouver les conditions physiologiques et expérimentales qui déterminent une accumulation de substance neurosécrétée au niveau des cellules nerveuses hypothalamiques et de leurs prolongements: il faut en deuxième lieu apporter la preuve que les chaînettes de grains que l'on peut observer en divers points de l'encéphale sont bien d'origine neurosécrétoire hypothalamique. Dès le début de nos travaux nous nous sommes préoccupés de rechercher les conditions favorables permettant la mise en évidence de ces voies, ce qui se trouve réalisé lorsqu'il existe une accumulation de substance neurosécrétée au niveau des éléments cellulaires des noyaux hypothalamiques; les axones de ces éléments cellulaires sont alors bien dessinés souvent sur de longs parcours; leurs terminaisons sont fréquemment marquées d'une façon manifeste par des chaînettes ou des chapelets de grains de taille variable.

Chez la Poule les conditions expérimentales qui réalisent cette accumulation de substance neurosécrétée sont représentées notamment par les injections d'extraits post-hypophysaires, d'oestrogène ou d'hormone thyréotrope. C'est principalement l'étude d'animaux soumis à des injections d'hormone thyréotrope qui nous a permis de décrire chez les Oiseaux des voies neurosécrétoires extra-hypothalamo-neurohypophysaires.

Chez les Batraciens les injections d'hormone thyréotrope et d'oestrogène augmentent également l'importance de la substance neurosécrétée au niveau des cellules des noyaux hypothalamiques (Triton et Grenouille); mais cette accumulation s'est révélée ici beaucoup moins manifeste que chez les Oiseaux, nous incitant à rechercher et à utiliser d'autres conditions expérimentales favorables. L'hypophysectomie totale chez la Grenouille détermine au niveau du tractus préoptico-hypophysaire une accumulation de substance chromo-hématoxylinophile; au fur et à mesure que l'on s'éloigne de la date de l'intervention, l'hématoxyline colore les fibres nerveuses de plus en plus près de leur origine; la substance chromo-hématoxylinophile s'accumule au niveau des cellules des noyaux hypothalamiques, des fibres neurosécrétoires extra-hypophysaires se manifestent. L'ablation du seul lobe glandulaire de l'hypophyse permet d'obtenir un résultat moindre que précédemment certes, mais suffisant pour l'étude de ces voies. L'énucléation bilatérale, seule ou associée à l'hypophysectomie totale ou partielle, l'ablation de la paraphyse sont des procédés opératoires qui facilitent cette étude.

Mais si ces diverses techniques sont aisées chez les Batraciens, elles sont d'application moins facile chez les autres Vertébrés; c'est pourquoi nous avons recherché une méthode plus simple et dont les résultats soient aussi constants que possible. Or, après divers essais, il est apparu que la mise en place des animaux aquatiques (Poissons-Batraciens) dans une solution de dextrose à 1, 5 à 3%, pendant deux à quatre jours se révélait suffisamment efficace. L'absorption forcée ou non d'une solution de dextrose à 5% a été utilisée chez les animaux terrestres; elle nous a donné un résultat satisfaisant chez les Reptiles et les Oiseaux, mais médiocre chez les Mammifères[1]. Il est certain que dans cette dernière

---

[1] Il est bon d'indiquer que des solutions plus concentrées (de 5 à 10%) sont en général mal supportées et déterminent un appauvrissement en substance neurosécrétée chez toutes les espèces.

classe des Vertébrés, si l'hibernation représente une condition physiologique favorable à l'étude de ces voies, les conditions expérimentales qui en permettraient une mise en évidence aisée restent encore à préciser; en effet, ni l'ingestion d'eau sucrée, ni l'injection d'hormone thyréotrope, de thyroxine ou d'oestrogène, procédés que nous avons utilisés (Souris, Rat, Hamster), n'apportent de résultats aussi favorables que chez les autres Vertébrés.

Afin de prouver la nature neurosécrétoire des chaînettes de grains observées nous avons fixé nos pièces soit dans le liquide de Bouin ou Bouin Hollande soit dans le formol ou l'alcool chloroforme; les préparations ont été colorées soit par l'hématoxyline chromique phloxine soit par la fuchsine paraldéhyde avec ou sans oxydation, soit par la méthode de Sloper au bleu Alcian.

Nous avons cherché par ailleurs à apporter une preuve expérimentale de la réalité de ces voies, en effectuant chez la Grenouille l'ablation de la paraphyse et en sectionnant chez la Tortue l'extrémité antérieure du télencéphale; ces interventions se sont accompagnées de résultats positifs que nous analyserons plus loin, qui sont en faveur de l'existence de voies au niveau de l'encéphale autres que la voie neurosécrétoire hypothalamo-neurohypophysaire.

Anatomie topographique et microscopique des voies neurosécrétoires extra-hypophysaires chez les Poissons

Il existe chez les Téléostéens étudiés (Truite, Carpe, Loche, Tanche) (Fig. 1), des caractéristiques communes; ces voies dans l'ensemble sont courtes. Les unes sont dirigées en avant vers le striatum. D'autres peuvent être suivies au voisinage ou le long des voies olfactives; de courtes fibres se dirigent vers les ganglions de l'habenula, mais contrairement à Stutinsky nous ne les avons jamais vu pénétrer dans ces formations. Le fait le plus curieux observé chez deux de ces espèces (Truite, Carpe), est la pénétration de fibres neurosécrétoires à l'intérieur des diverses parties glandulaires de l'hypophyse. Elles sont évidentes dans la pars intermedia où elles se

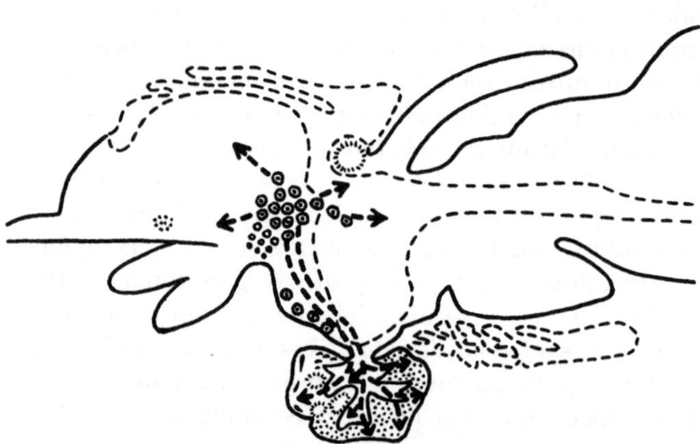

Fig. 1. Schéma représentant les voies hypothalamo-extra-neurohypophysaires chez *Salmo irideus* (coupe sagittale du cerveau; l'extrémité antérieure est à gauche). Sont indiquées les voies hypothalamostriatale et habénulaire; en bas le tractus hypothalamo-neurohypophysaire montre des terminaisons dans la pars intermedia (en arrière) et dans la zone glandulaire moyenne (en avant)

terminent fréquemment au contact des cellules chromophobes intermédiaires. Elles sont nombreuses dans la région glandulaire moyenne correspondant à la pars distalis des Vertébrés supérieurs où ces fibres paraissent se terminer comme l'a déjà constaté da Lage (1955) chez l'Hippocampe au contact des seules cellules cyanophiles (ces dernières se colorent chez les Téléostéens d'une façon beaucoup plus intense par l'hématoxyline chromique que dans les autres classes des Vertébrés); nous n'avons jusqu'à présent jamais observé de terminaisons indéniables au contact des cellules éosinophiles; ces fibres neurosécrétoires existent également quoique peu nombreuses dans la partie folliculaire de l'organe.

Ces terminaisons neurosécrétoires au niveau de la partie glandulaire de l'hypophyse sont extrêmement nettes chez les Téléostéens étudiés. Malgré de nombreuses investigations, semblables recherches se sont avérées vaines chez les autres Vertébrés. On peut se demander si cette particularité morphologique est à rapprocher du fait que ces espèces possèdent une vascularisation particulière du complexe hypophysaire.

Anatomie topographique et microscopique des voies neurosécrétoires extra-hypophysaires chez les Batraciens

De même que chez les Téléostéens, il existe chez les Batraciens un plan général d'organisation de ces voies; mais nous trouvons cependant des différences entre Urodèles et Anoures qui nécessitent une description particulière pour chacun de ces groupes.

Chez les Urodèles (Fig. 2), dont le système nerveux parmi les Batraciens est le plus primitif, la voie neurosécrétoire la plus évidente et la plus facile à observer est assez courte et para-médiane; des deux noyaux préoptiques s'échappent de nombreuses fibres colorées sur de longs parcours qui se dirigent en avant vers la région septale et plus particulièrement vers une région épendymaire située sur la ligne médiane dont nous avons précisé auparavant les caractères et qui est l'homologue de l'organe subfornical des Mammi-

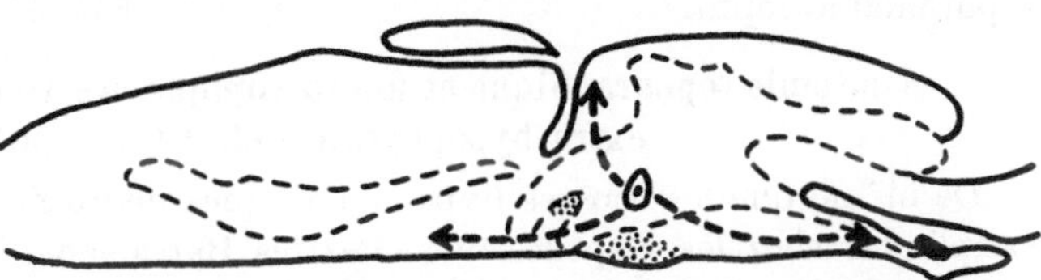

Fig. 2. Schéma représentant les voies hypothalamo-extra-neurohypophysaires chez *Triturus alpestris* (coupe sagittale du cerveau; l'extrémité antérieure est à gauche). De haut en bas et à gauche, sont indiquées successivement les voies hypothalamo-habénulaire, septale et télencéphalique; à droite, le tractus hypothalamo-neurohypophysaire

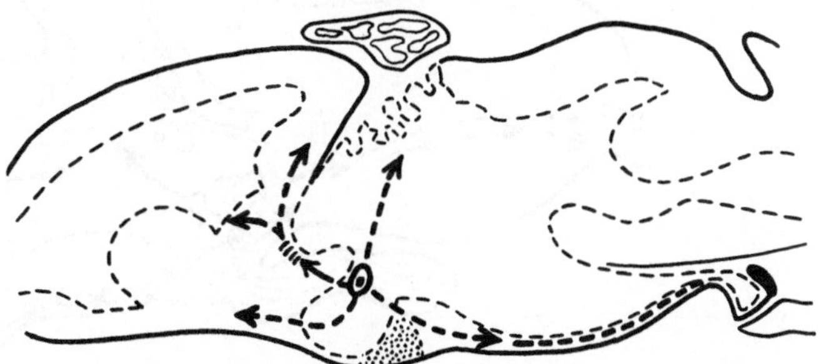

Fig. 3. Schéma représentant les voies hypothalamo-extra-neurohypophysaires chez *Rana esculenta* (coupe sagittale du cerveau; l'extrémité antérieure est à gauche). De haut en bas et à gauche sont indiquées successivement les voies hypothalamo-habénulaire, septale et hippocampique, télencéphalique; à droite le tractus hypothalamo-neurohypophysaire

fères. Cette voie est certainement une des plus manifestes; nous verrons qu'elle présente les mêmes caractères d'évidence chez toutes les espèces étudiées.

Une voie ascendante hypothalamo-sous-habénulaire paire peut être observée; mais les fibres neurosécrétoires qui la constituent paraissent se terminer sur les faces latérales des noyaux de l'habénula; aucune fibre neurosécrétoire n'a pu en effet être observée chez les Urodèles à l'intérieur de ces noyaux, alors qu'il est facile de les observer chez la Grenouille, la plupart des Reptiles étudiés et les Oiseaux.

Des fibres neurosécrétoires peuvent être observées principalement de part et d'autre de la scissure interhémisphérique à la partie inférieure du cerveau antérieur représentant une voie hypothalamo-télencéphalique dont quelques éléments peuvent être suivis jusqu'au voisinage de l'extrémité postérieure des ventricules latéraux.

Chez les Anoures (Fig. 3), nous retrouvons les mêmes voies hypothalamo-septales et hypothalamo-habénulaires; les premières se terminant également au voisinage d'une région épendymaire homologue de l'organe subfornical placée également en position ventrale au niveau de l'espace interventriculaire. Par ailleurs, un certain nombre de fibres paraissent aboutir aux noyaux de la commissure hippocampique[1] et à ceux de la racine de la commissure palliale. Les voies hypothalamo-télencéphaliques sont plus courtes que chez les Urodèles.

Il existe par conséquent des différences marquées entre Urodèles et Anoures. Dans ce dernier groupe, les fibres neurosécrétoires extra-hypophysaires colorées apparaissent constamment plus nombreuses, principalement le long de la voie hypothalamo-septale.

Anatomie topographique et microscopique des voies neurosécrétoires extra-hypophysaires chez les Reptiles

De même que les centres hypothalamiques neurosécrétoires apparaissent plus compliqués chez les Reptiles que chez les Batraciens, les voies neurosécrétoires extra-hypophysaires présentent une complexité plus grande. Relativement

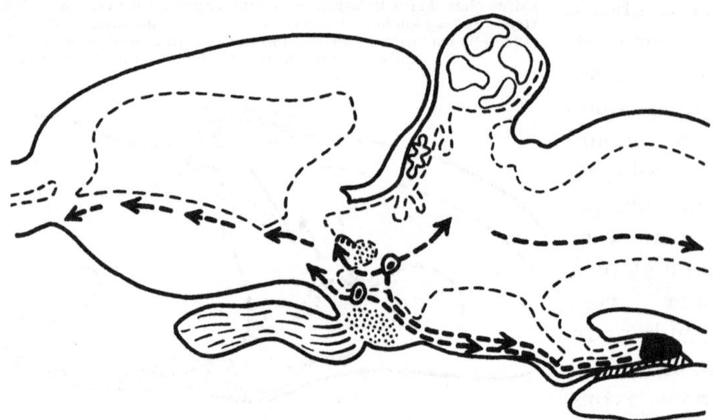

Fig. 4. Schéma représentant les voies hypothalamo-extra-neurohypophysaires chez *Testudo mauritanica* (coupe sagittale du cerveau; l'extrémité antérieure est à gauche). De haut en bas et à gauche, sont indiquées successivement les voies hypothalamo-habénulaire, septale et télencéphalique; à droite et en haut, l'orientation générale des fibres neurosécrétoires postérieures; à droite et en bas le tractus hypothalamo-neurohypophysaire

simples encore chez la Tortue dont le système nerveux central représente un des types les moins évolués, elles paraissent beaucoup plus complexes chez le Lézard et surtout chez les Serpents étudiés.

Chez la Tortue (Fig. 4), nous retrouvons les mêmes voies hypothalamo-septales (l'homologue de l'organe subfornical est là encore en position ventrale) et hypothalamo-habénulaires. Mais ce qui caractérise cette espèce, c'est l'importance de

---

[1] Elles sont particulièrement nombreuses après ablation de la paraphyse et aboutissent à la racine de cet organe; elles paraissent lui être destinées.

la voie hypothalamo-télencéphalique; celle-ci est particulièrement longue, puisque après avoir longé les ventricules latéraux, elle gagne l'extrémité antérieure du cerveau et atteint le lobe olfactif. La réalité de cette longue voie nous paraît expérimentalement démontrée: après section de l'extrémité antérieure du télencéphale chez cette espèce, on constate en effet l'accumulation de substance neurosécrétée immédiatement en arrière de la tranche de section. Par ailleurs, il existe en avant du chiasma et sous le récessus optique, de part et d'autre de la ligne médiane un nombre important de fibres neurosécrétoires qui gagnent la face inférieure du télencéphale en s'écartant de chaque coté de la partie postéro-inférieure de la scissure interhémisphérique. Ce faisceau numériquement important paraît représenter une voie hypothalamo-télencéphalique inférieure. Quelques fibres neurosécrétoires peuvent être également observées le long de l'aqueduc de

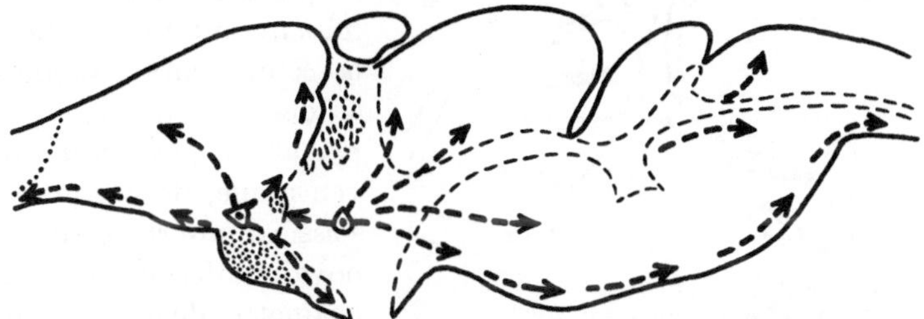

Fig. 5. Schéma représentant les voies hypothalamo-extra-neurohypophysaires chez *Natrix natrix* (coupe sagittale du cerveau; l'extrémité antérieure est à gauche, l'hypophyse n'est pas figurée). De haut en bas et à gauche, sont indiquées successivement les voies hypothalamo-habénulaire septale, palliale et télencéphalique; à droite, l'orientation et l'importance des fibres neurosécrétoires postérieures

Sylvius; ces fibres postérieures paraissent peu importantes chez la Tortue; nous verrons qu'elles sont beaucoup plus développées chez le Lézard et la Couleuvre.

Chez le Lézard, nous trouvons les mêmes voies neurosécrétoires; mais il existe d'autre part des chaînettes de grains en direction de la commissure palliale postérieure et d'autres vers la commissure postérieure et l'organe sous-commissural; des fibres neurosécrétoires plus nombreuses peuvent être enfin observées au niveau du plancher du quatrième ventricule et dans la région ventrale du bulbe.

Chez la Couleuvre (Fig. 5), l'importance des voies neurosécrétoires est encore plus manifeste. Les voies télencéphaliques, septales et habénulaires peuvent être retrouvées; mais également des fibres en direction du néostriatum, de la commissure palliale postérieure et enfin de la commissure postérieure et de l'organe sous-commissural; d'autres fibres peuvent être aisément observées au contact ou à l'intérieur des éléments de l'organe paraventriculaire et de l'épendyme du troisième ventricule. Les fibres postérieures chez cette espèce sont également nombreuses; quelques-unes pénètrent la substance réticulée du mésencéphale; d'autres longent la face ventrale du mésencéphale et du bulbe; mais le plus grand nombre se termine au voisinage de l'épendyme de l'aqueduc de Sylvius et du plancher du 4° ventricule.

Anatomie topographique et microscopique des voies neurosécrétoires extra-hypophysaires chez les Oiseaux

Les voies efférentes neurosécrétoires extra-neurohypophysaires que nous avons pu observer chez plusieurs espèces d'Oiseaux, sont extrêmement nettes;

au nombre de deux à trajet ascendant, elles peuvent être mises en évidence chez la Poule (Fig. 6), contrairement à la voie classique descendante, sur tout leur parcours; celui-ci est en effet dessiné soit par des fibres bien colorées par l'hématoxyline chromique, soit par de nombreuses chaînettes de grains neurosécrétés qui suivent les trajets fibrillaires.

De ces deux voies, l'une hypothalamo-septale est d'observation facile; elle prend son origine au niveau de la partie pré-optique du noyau supra-optique et au niveau des cellules antérieures du noyau paraventriculaire. Les fibres d'origine préoptique se dirigent vers le noyau de la commissure palliale en passant en avant de la commissure antérieure. Les fibres d'origine paraventriculaire atteignent ce noyau en passant en arrière de la commissure antérieure. Le noyau de la commissure palliale est situé au-dessus de la commissure palliale, en avant du toit du 3° ventricule, de chaque côté de la scissure interhémisphérique. Ce noyau renferme constamment des chaînettes de grains neurosécrétés toujours très nombreuses. Quelques-unes se dirigent vers la paroi épendymaire avoisinante, d'autres se terminent au contact des capillaires de cette région, d'autres se mettent en rapport avec les cellules nerveuses de ce noyau. Mais un grand nombre

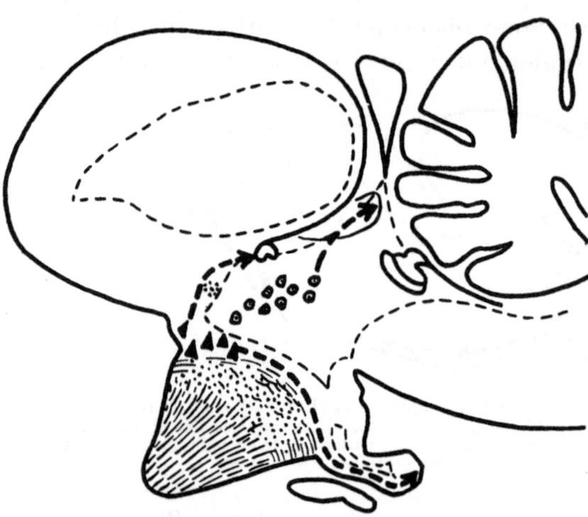

Fig. 6. Schéma représentant les voies hypothalamo-extra-neurohypophysaires chez *Gallus domesticus* (coupe sagittale du cerveau; l'extrémité antérieure est à gauche). D'avant en arrière sont indiquées en haut les voies hypothalamo-septale et habénulaire, en bas le tractus hypothalamo-neurohypophysaire

d'entre elles poursuivent leur chemin vers le pied de l'organe subfornical et se terminent à l'intérieur de ce petit organe où elles ne sont visibles que dans certaines conditions physiologiques (ponte) et expérimentales (injections de T. S. H.).

L'autre voie ascendante, dont l'étude est plus difficile, est hypothalamo-habénulaire. Les cellules les plus dorsales et postérieures du noyau paraventriculaire sont en relation par leurs axones avec les noyaux de l'habénula où se rencontrent un grand nombre de chaînettes chez tous les Oiseaux étudiés (Canard, Pigeon, Moineau, Gros-Bec). Il est possible que quelques fibres neurosécrétoires venant du noyau de la commissure palliale suivent le tractus septo-habénulaire et se terminent également au niveau des ganglions habénulaires. Au niveau de ces derniers les chaînettes peuvent soit se terminer au contact des grandes cellules nerveuses des noyaux habénulaires ou se mêler aux fibres de la strie médullaire.

Anatomie topographique et microscopique des voies neurosécrétoires extra-hypophysaires chez les Mammifères

L'objet le plus favorable pour l'étude de ces voies dans cette classe de Vertébrés, ainsi que l'a montré Barry est certainement la Chauve-Souris en hibernation. En particulier chez le Rhinolophe (objet que nous avons pu également étudier), cet auteur a décrit plusieurs de ces voies: une voie hypothalamo-épithalamique (noyau paratoenial) et épiphysaire, une voie hypothalamo-mésencéphalique, une voie postérieure hypothalamo-protubérantielle et bulbaire, enfin des voies antérieures hypothalamo-rhinencéphaliques et latérales hypothalamo-latéro-ventriculaires. Ces recherches que cet auteur s'est efforcé d'étendre à d'autres Mammifères, se sont révélées assez décevantes; nous-mêmes chez le Rat, la Souris et le Hamster commun ou doré placés en diverses conditions expérimentales (ingestion d'eau sucrée, injections d'oestrogène, d'hormone thyréotrope ou de thyroxine) n'avons obtenu que des résultats fragmentaires. Chez le Hamster (Fig. 7 et 8), cependant, nous avons pu mettre en évidence des fibres neurosécrétoiresantérieures hypothalamo-rhinencéphaliques et latérales s'étendant jusqu'aux

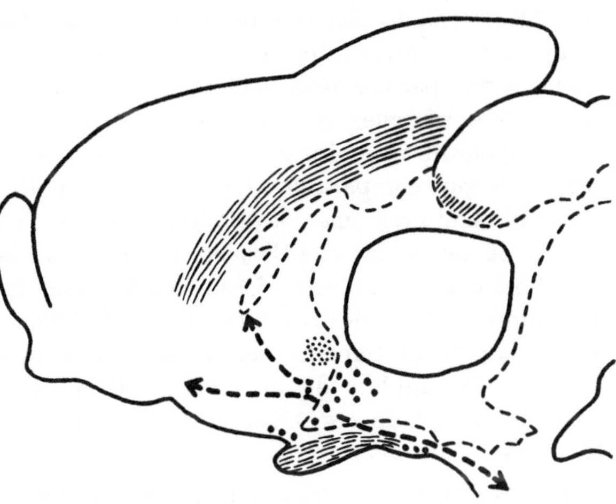

Fig. 7. Schéma représentant les voies hypothalamo-extra-neurohypophysaires chez *Cricetus auratus* (coupe sagittale du cerveau; l'extrémité antérieure est à gauche). D'avant en arrière sont indiquées en haut les voies hypothalamo-télencéphaliques et juxtaventriculaires; en bas, le tractus hypothalamo-neurohypophysaire

parois du ventricule latéral et en direction du corps strié[1]. Il nous semble d'après ces résultats que les conditions d'étude physiologiques et expérimentales de ces voies neurosécrétoires doivent être à nouveau envisagées; seuls comptent

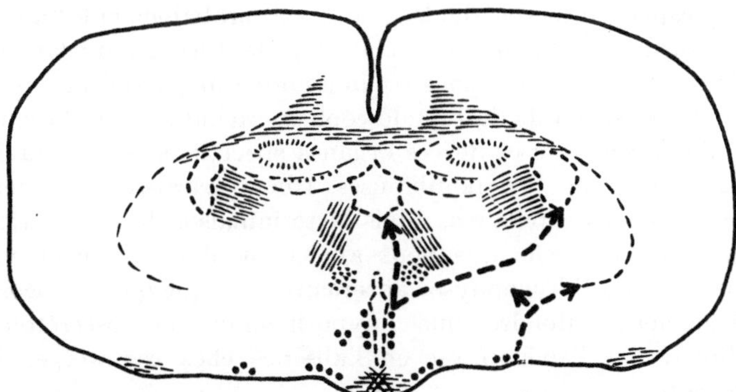

Fig. 8. Coupe frontale du Cerveau passant en arrière de la commissure antérieure chez *Cricetus auratus* montrant l'orientation des voies neurosécrétoires hypothalamo-medio-et latero-ventriculaires et celle des fibres se dirigeant vers le corps strié

les résultats positifs et ceux obtenus par BARRY chez les Chauves-Souris et que nous avons pu vérifier, laissent entendre que ces voies neurosécrétoires extra-hypothalamo-neurohypophysaires sont chez les Mammifères plus étendues que ne le font penser nos observations.

---

[1] Des fibres existent également au voisinage du ventricule médian représentant peut-être l'homologue de la voie hypothalamo-septale qui est manifeste chez les autres Vertébrés.

Discussion

Il existe par conséquent dans la série des Vertébrés des voies neurosécrétoires hypothalamiques extra-neurohypophysaires, mises en évidence par des chaînettes de grains neurosécrétés, qui suivent les trajets fibrillaires, quelquefois par de véritables corps de Herring, dont les caractéristiques sont identiques à celles de la substance neurosécrétée et distinctes de la substance chromo-hématoxylinophile élaborée par certaines cellules nerveuses, les cellules névrogliques ou épendymaires. Il existe chez les différentes espèces des différences notables, mais cependant il apparaît au moins chez les Vertébrés inférieurs et les Sauropsidés un plan d'organisation comparable. Les voies hypothalamo-septales et habénulaires sont rudimentaires chez les Poissons et les Urodèles mais bien développées chez les Anoures, les Reptiles et les Oiseaux. Les voies neurosécrétoires télencéphaliques sont rudimentaires chez les Poissons et les Batraciens, mais bien développées chez les Reptiles et probablement les Mammifères. Mais ces premières constatations ne permettent pas cependant de conclure en raison des caractères incomplets de nos recherches chez les Oiseaux et les Mammifères si la complexité de ces voies va de pair avec le développement de l'encéphale dans la série des Vertébrés.

Il n'est naturellement pas facile d'indiquer comment se terminent ces fibres même en associant une imprégnation argentique à une coloration à la fuchsine paraldéhyde. La terminaison de ces fibres au contact de cellules nerveuses ou gliales est probable; mais les images observées à ce propos sont rarement indiscutables. Il est nécessaire de souligner, d'autre part, l'importance des fibres se terminant au contact de l'épithélium épendymaire des ventricules latéraux, du troisième ventricule et de ses organes spécialisés du 3° ventricule. Elles sont chez les Batraciens principalement nettes au niveau de cette région vascularisée située au niveau de l'espace interventriculaire qui est probablement l'homologue de l'organe subfornical des Mammifères, chez les Reptiles au niveau de l'organe paraventriculaire et de l'organe sous-commissural qui participent certainement à l'élaboration de constituants du liquide céphalo-rachidien. Ces faits impliquent que l'activité de l'épendyme et de ces organes spécialisés est liée indirectement au métabolisme de l'eau. De nombreuses fibres paraissent se terminer au contact de la paroi des capillaires. Mais la terminaison la plus curieuse observée, après DA LAGE, est celle que nous avons pu observer au niveau des éléments cyanophiles de l'hypophyse antérieure de quelques Téléostéens. Ce fait laisse également entendre que l'hypothalamus neurosécrétoire possède une action directe sur l'adénophyse en l'absence chez ces espèces de système porte-hypophysaire.

Cependant un grand nombre de ces fibres après avoir perdu ses propriétés tinctoriales disparaît sans qu'on puisse indiquer avec certitude leur mode de terminaison. Les méthodes que nous avons utilisées, si elles permettent de topographier avec assez de bonheur ces voies hypothalamo-extraneuro-hypophysaires et d'affirmer qu'elles ne représentent pas des fibres aberrantes du faisceau hypothalamo-neurohypophysaire, méritent cependant d'être améliorées pour étendre encore nos connaissances au sujet des relations de l'hypothalamus neurosécrétoire avec les autres parties du système nerveux central.

Bibliographie

ANANTHANARAYANAN, V.: Nature and distribution of neurosecretory cells of the reptilian brain. Z. Zellforsch. **43**, 8 (1955).

BARGMANN, W.: Neurosekretion und hypothalamisch-hypophysäres System. Verh. anat. Ges. **100**, 30 (1953).

BARRY, J.: De l'existence de voies neurosécrétoires hypothalamo-télencéphaliques chez la Chauve-souris (Rhinolophus ferrum equinum) et état d'hibernation. Bull. Soc. Sci. Nancy **13**, 126 (1954).

— Etude de la neurosécrétion diencéphalique chez la Chauve-souris en état d'hibernation. C. R. Ass. Anat. Gênes, 41° réunion 179 (1954).

— Les voies extra-hypophysaires de la neurosécrétion diencéphalique. C. R. Ass. Anat. Paris, 42° réunion, 264 (1955).

DA LAGE, C.: Innervation neurosécrétoire de l'adénohypophyse chez l'Hippocampe. C. R. Ass. Anat. Gênes, 41° réunion 361 (1954).

— Etude supravitale de l'hypophyse de l'Hippocampe en microscopie à contraste de phase. C. R. Ass. Anat. Paris, 42° réunion, 1954 (1955).

HILD, W.: Vergleichende Untersuchungen über Neurosekretion im Zwischenhirn von Amphibien und Reptilien. Z. Anat. **115**, 459 (1951).

LEGAIT, H.: Etude histophysiologique et expérimentale du système hypothalamo-neurohypophysaire de la Poule Rhode-Island. Arch. Anat. micr. Morph. exp. **44**, 323 (1955).

— Les voies efférentes des noyaux neurosécrétoires hypothalamiques chez les Oiseaux. C. R. Soc. Biol. (Paris) **150**, 996 (1956).

— Anatomie microscopique des noyaux hypothalamiques neurosécrétoires et de leurs voies efférentes chez la Poule Rhode-Island. Acta neuroveg. (Wien) **15**, 252 (1957).

— et E. LEGAIT: Mise en évidence de voies neurosécrétoires extra-hypothalamo-hypophysaires chez quelques Batraciens et Reptiles. C. R. Soc. Biol. (Paris) **150**, 1429 (1956).

— et E. LEGAIT: A propos de la structure et de l'innervation des organes épendymaires du troisième ventricule chez les Batraciens et les Reptiles. C. R. Soc. Biol. (Paris) **150**, 1982 (1956).

SCHARRER, E.: Neurosecretion X. A relationship between the paraphysis and the paraventricular nucleus in the garter snake (Thamnophis Sp.). Biol. Bull. (Lancaster) **101**, 106 (1951).

STUTINSKY, F.: Contribution à l'étude du complexe hypothalamo-hypophysaire. Thèse, Fac. Sciences. Paris 1955.

Department of Pharmacology of the University of Milan, Italy

Neurosecretion and Stimulation of the Adenohypophysis

By

L. MARTINI

A great deal of evidence indicates that the release of pituitary adrenocortico-trophic (ACTH), somatotrophic (STH) and thyrotrophic (TSH) hormones is under hypothalamic control.

This conclusion has been supported by experiments in which portions of the hypothalamus have been either stimulated or destroyed, and by experiments involving the severance of the pituitary stalk and or transplantation of the pituitary gland to a site remote from the *sella turcica* [HARRIS (1955)].

The view that hypophyseal portal vessels regulate anterior pituitary function by transmitting a hypothalamic humoral substance, has received support from the results of several anatomical and physiological studies.

In confirmation of earlier observations WORTHINGTON (1955) has recently shown that blood in the portal vessels of the mouse flows from the capillaries in the *median eminence* to the sinusoids of the *pars distalis*.

There is little doubt that the neurosecretory material stainable with Gomori's chrome-alum-hematoxylin and phloxin and present in the neurohypophysis may be depleted by noxious stimuli of the sort which are also known to induce the release of ACTH [ROTHBALLER (1953), SCHARRER et al. (1954)]. These findings are compatible with the view that a component of neurosecretory material, liberated by the nerve endings in the median eminence and infundibular stem, can be carried via the portal vessels into the *pars distalis* of the pituitary to affect the activity of this gland.

Several suggestions have been put forward as to the nature of the component of neurosecretory material which could stimulate the adenohypophysis. In recent years attention was drawn to a possible relationship between the antidiuretic hormone (ADH) of the posterior pituitary system and ACTH secretion. This view was mainly based on the demonstration that extracts containing ADH are effective in inducing ACTH release in normal animals [MARTINI (1957)], in hypo-physectomized animals bearing a functional pituitary graft in the anterior chamber of the eye [MARTINI et al. (1956)], and in rats with hypothalamic lesions which block the response to non-specific stimuli [McCANN et al. (1954)]. Recently the ACTH-releasing activity of posterior pituitary extracts has been confirmed in an *in vitro* system but here the activity of these extracts has been ascribed to the presence of a contaminant [SAFFRAN et al. (1955)].

It seemed of interest to reinvestigate *in vivo* the effect of different substances, known to occur in certain hypothalamic neurones, on the ACTH releasing mechanism, using normal rats, hypophysectomized rats, hypophysectomized rats bearing a functional pituitary graft in the anterior chamber of the eye, and rats in which the ACTH discharge resulting from noxious stimuli had been blocked by previous administration of 9-α-fluoro-hydrocortisone.

In normal rats the intraperitoneal injection of adrenaline, noradrenaline, acetylcholine, histamine, serotonin, Pitressin (ADH, Parke-Davis), Pitocin (oxytocic hormone, Parke-Davis) and of a preparation of synthetic oxytocin was followed by a highly significant fall in adrenal ascorbic acid concentration. Two different samples of substance P (kindly supplied by Professor GADDUM and by Professor VON EULER) were completely ineffective in the ascorbic acid depletion test.

Pitressin and Pitocin were ineffective in the hypophysectomized rats, thus showing that they were not contaminated with ACTH.

In the rats containing grafts, the local application of acetylcholine, histamine, serotonin, Pitocin and synthetic oxytocin was completely ineffective; adrenaline gave a small response in some rats, but this result cannot be considered as significant. Among the drugs tested, only Pitressin gave a significant fall in adrenal ascorbic acid concentration, when directly applied to the grafted pituitary gland.

In the steroid-inhibited rats the intravenous administration of the different "stressors" was completely ineffective; only Pitressin could overcome the blockade; the result obtained with Pitocin was much less significant.

Intracarotid administration of very small doses of Pitressin are still active in the "blocked" rats; in these rats Pitressin gives a linear log-dose relationship in doses ranging from 0,1 to 0,4 micrograms.

In "blocked" rats the intracarotid injection of hypertonic saline solution (NaCl 2%), a very effective ADH releaser [VERNEY (1946)], produces a very marked fall in adrenal ascorbic acid.

These experiments suggest that a neurohumoral substance which stimulates the release of ACTH by acting directly at the hypophyseal level is present in posthypophyseal extracts, but do not allow one to conclude about its nature; in particular they do not exclude that the effect observed after Pitressin administration could in part be due to a contaminant with specific ACTH-releasing properties (SAFFRAN's Cortico-Releasing-Factor-CRF). It should however be pointed out that it has recently been demonstrated that synthetic lysine-vasopressin has an ACTH stimulating activity, both *in vivo* and *in vitro* [McDONALD et al. (1956), SAFFRAN et al. (1957)]. SAFFRAN (1957) himself states that synthetic lysine-vasopressin is active in his modified *in vitro* method at a dose level of 5 millimicrograms and that his most purified CRF preparation is only 10 times as potent as lysine-vasopressin in this system.

The results of the present study as well as SAFFRAN's (1957) and McDONALD's (1956) results could suggest that the stimulation of ACTH release, from a physiological point of view, could be evoked through the release of both factors: SAFFRAN's CRF and vasopressin.

It was then investigated whether the same hypothalamic mediators which regulate the release of ACTH from the anterior pituitary could also stimulate the release of somatotrophic and thyrotrophic hormones.

The following results were obtained:

A chronic treatment with the extract of a whole posterior pituitary or with a more purified ADH preparation (Pitressin, Parke-Davis) induces, both in male and female normal rats, a statistically significant enlargement of the epiphyseal cartilage width. The lack of such an effect in the hypophysectomized animals supports the view that the stimulus to the tibia cartilage plate is due to an activation of the STH secretion by the pituitary.

The intraperitoneal injection of Pitressin into normal, but not into hypophysectomized rats, is followed by a stimulation of thyroid I_{131} uptake; the intravenous injection of Pitressin into normal rabbits produces a marked elevation of TSH blood levels, as measured by Bottari's (1956) method.

References

Bottari, P.: Arch. int. Physiol. **64**, 117 (1956).

Harris, G. W.: Neural Control of the Pituitary Gland. London: Edward Arnold Ltd. 1955.

Martini, L., and A. De Poli: J. Endocr. **13**, 229 (1956).

— Fisiopatologia del Diencefalo. Berlin: Springer (in press).

McCann, S. M., and J. R. Brobeck: Proc. Soc. exp. Biol. (N. Y.) **87**, 318 (1954).

McDonald, K. K., V. R. Weise and R. W. Patrick: Proc. Soc. exp. Biol. (N. Y.) **93**, 348 (1956).

Rothballer, A. B.: Anat. Rec. **115**, 21 (1953).

Saffran, M., A. V. Schally and B. G. Benfey: Endocrinology **57**, 439 (1955).

— — The End. Soc., p. 102. 39th Meetg. (1957).

Scharrer, E.: Fifth Annual Report on Stress, p. 185. New York: M. D. Publications Inc. 1955.

— and R. D. Frandson: Anat. Rec. **118**, 350 (1954).

Verney, E. B.: Lancet **2**, 781 (1946).

Worthington, W. C.: Bull. Johns Hopk. Hosp. **97**, 343 (1955).

Allan Memorial Institute of Psychiatry, McGill University, Montreal, Canada

Characterization of the Corticotrophin Releasing Factor of the Neurohypophysis

By

M. SAFFRAN, A. V. SCHALLY*, M. SEGAL** and B. ZIMMERMANN

With 5 Figures

The mammalian hypothalamic-neurohypophysial neurosecretory system produces and releases two potent agents, vasopressin and oxytocin, which exert powerful actions on other organs of the animal. These hormones are peptides composed of 8 amino acids arranged like the figure 9 in a ring of 5 amino acids and a tail of 3 amino acids (Fig. 1). Oxytocin differs from vasopressin in only 2 of the amino acids.

Oxytocin and vasopressin are prepared commercially by separation from posterior lobe powder. The first steps in the procedure (Table 1) remove the water, fat and larger proteins. The residue consists largely of a mixture of peptides and small proteins. Chromatography on filter paper resolves this mixture into a series of fractions (Fig. 2), which can be visualized by spraying with ninhydrin. The area between the markers of lysine and glycine contain vasopressin and oxytocin. The other

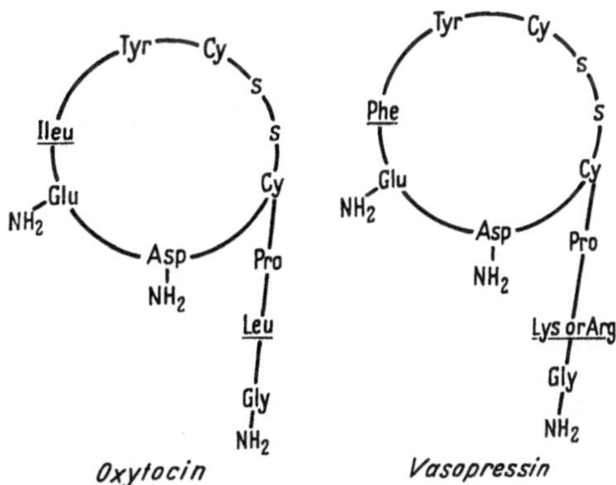

Fig. 1. Chemical structure of Oxytocin and Vasopressin. *Gly* glycine; *Leu* leucine; *Pro* proline; *Cy-S-S-Cy* cystine; *Tyr* tyrosine; *Ileu* isoleucine; *Glu* glutamic acid; *Asp* aspartic acid; *Phe* phenylalanine; *Lys* lysine; *Arg* arginine. NH_2 terminal amino or amide groups. The underlined amino acids indicate the positions that differ in the hormones

zones are amino compounds of unknown biological activities. How many of these zones contain substances with potent biological effects, and how many represent products of the neurosecretory cells?

Our studies have been focussed on the detection and identification of the hypothalamic neurohumor postulated to control the release of corticotrophin (ACTH) from the adenohypophysis (2). The system used to detect the corticotrophin-releasing factor (CRF) is outlined in Fig. 3. Anterior pituitary tissue of the rat, represented by the bilobed structure at the top of the figure, is cut into two equal parts, which are incubated separately in bicarbonate buffered-

---

* Present address, Department of Physiology, Baylor University College of Medicine, Texas Medical Center, Houston, Texas.

** Elizabeth Holcombe Fellow.

Ringer medium. Both halves release ACTH into the medium. If nothing is added
to either half, then both halves release the same amount of ACTH (left side of

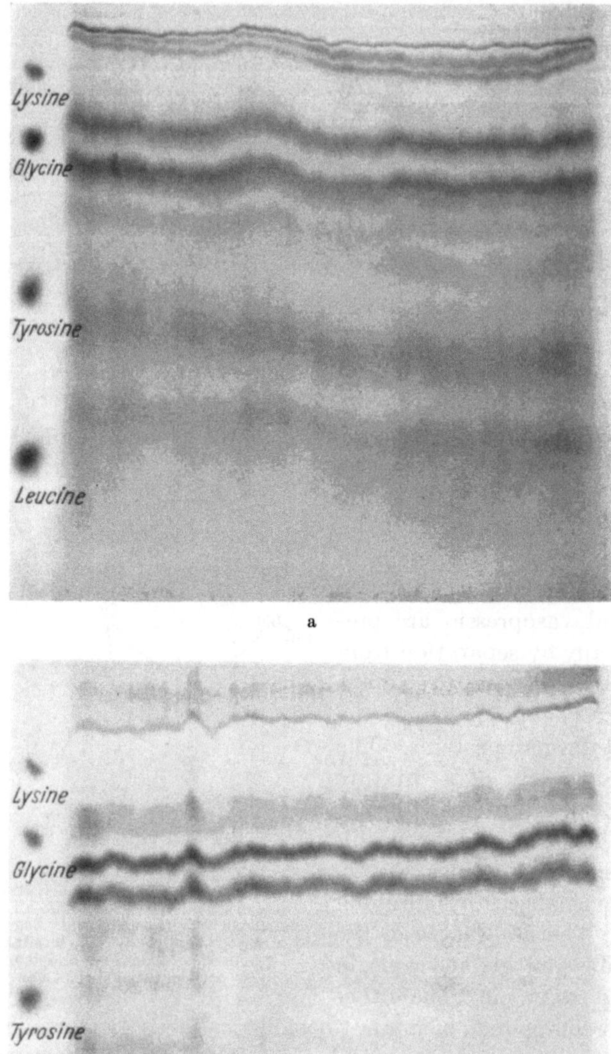

Fig. 2. Paper chromatography of Protopituitrin, Parke-Davis and Co. (a) and CRF-15, N. V. Organon (b)
in Butanol-acetic acid-water. The amino acids, lysine, glycine, tyrosine, and leucine, are used as marker
substances in this system

Fig. 3), while adding CRF to one of the halves results in a ratio > 1, in this case 3:1 (right side of Fig. 3) (*1, 3, 5, 6*). The ACTH is measured by an assay based upon the ability to stimulate the production of corticoids by rat adrenal glands *in vitro* (*4*).

Using this as a test system, the purification of CRF by paper chromatography could be followed. Fig. 4 illustrates the separation of CRF, shown by the shaded area, from a posterior pituitary concentrate, called "Protopituitrin", by *Parke-*

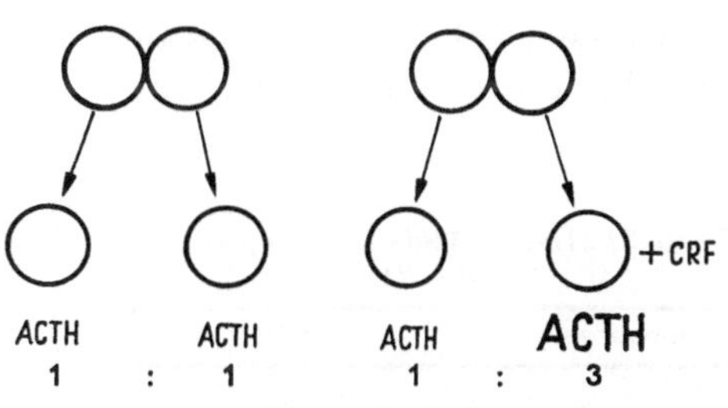

Fig. 3. *In vitro* test for CRF using the rat adenohypophysis

Davis, or CRF-15, by *Organon*. The preparation of this concentrate from posterior lobe powders is outlined in Table 1. Fig. 4, also demonstrates the positions that would be occupied by ACTH, vasopressin and oxytocin

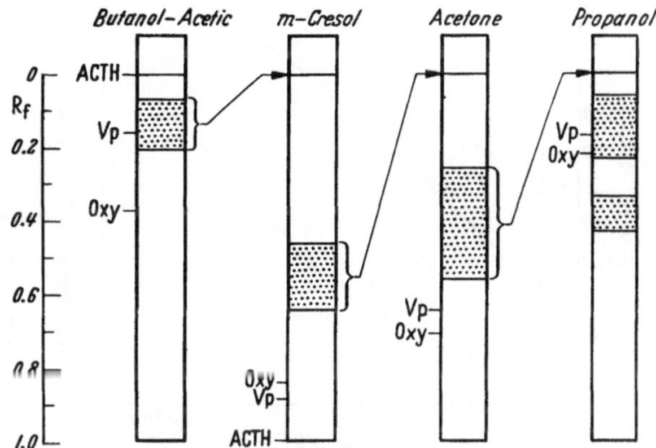

Fig. 4. Purification of CRF by serial chromatography, starting with Protopituitrin, which is first applied at $R_f = 0$ in the Butanol-Acetic system. ACTH, Vp and Oxy indicate the R_f's of corticotrophin, vasopressin and oxytocin respectively in each of the systems

in each of the chromatographic systems, and serves to indicate how CRF is completely separated from the other known hormones after chromatography in the first two systems.

Table 1. *Preparation of Posterior Pituitary Hormone Concentrate, Protopituitrin, Parke- Davis and Co., or CRF-15, N. V. Organon*

1. Extract posterior lobe acetone powder with hot 1/2% acetic acid.
2. Precipitate with ammonium sulfate.
3. Extract with glacial acetic acid.
4. Precipitate with ether and petroleum ether = CRF-15 or Protopituitrin.

The potencies of the preparations of CRF are judged by the smallest dose that significantly increases the release of ACTH in the test system. As outlined in Table 2, the consistent minimal effective dose of the starting material, Protopituitrin, is of the order of 10 micrograms. That of the most pure preparation, chromatographed 5 times in 4 separate systems, is of the order of 1 millimicrogram, a purification factor

Table 2. *Purification of CRF*

Fraction	R_f	Minimal dose micrograms
Protopituitrin		10.0
BuOH : HOAc : H₂O	0.05—0.20	2.5
m-Cresol : H₂O	0.46—0.64	0.3
m-Cresol : H₂O (Rechromatographed)	0.46—0.64	0.006
Acetone : H₂O	0.35—0.46	0.004
Propanol : H₂O	0.07—0.22	Approx. 0.001
	0.33—0.44	<0.001

of about 10,000. In various preparations the purification has ranged from 4,000 to 10,000-fold.

The stimulation of ACTH-release by CRF is roughly proportional to the log-dose (Fig. 5). The extent of the stimulation varies from experiment to experiment and, as illustrated in Fig. 5, the same preparation yields both positive and negative results at the 1.2 milli-microgram dose level in 2 separate experiments, thus demonstrating the necessity of repeated testing to establish the activity of a preparation.

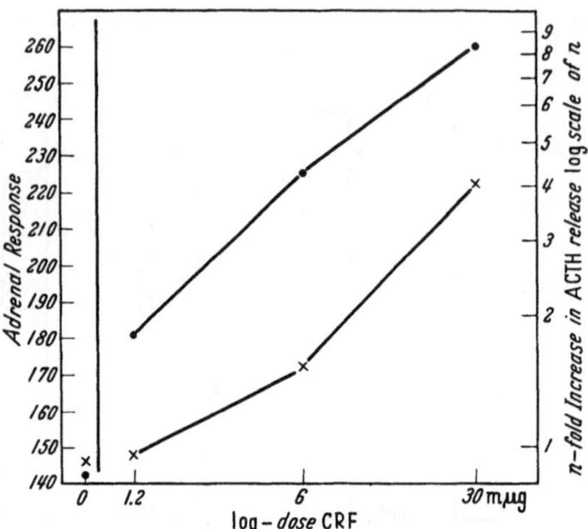

Fig. 5. Dose-response relationship of a CRF preparation at the second m-cresol stage, in two separate experiments. The left ordinate is in arbitrary units of adrenal response; the right ordinate is in terms of stimulation of the release of ACTH

Table 3. *Amino Acids in Vasopressin and CRF*

Vasopressin	CRF
Cystine	Cystine or Cysteine
Phenylalanine	Phenylalanine
Tyrosine	Tyrosine (trace)
Aspartic Acid	Aspartic Acid
Glutamic Acid	Glutamic Acid
Proline	Proline
Pysine or Arginine	Lysine
Glycine	Glycine
	Serine
	Histidine
	Alanine (trace)

Acid hydrolysis and chromatographic identification of the amino acids of potent CRF preparations has yielded the amino acids listed in Table 3. The identity of the amino acids varies slightly in the various preparations, as different impurities, or perhaps different CRF's, are included in the samples taken for

Table 4. *Biological Properties of Neurohypophysial Hormones*

Activity	Oxytocin	Beef Vasopressin	Hog Vasopressin	CRF
CRF (Minimal dose, mμg)	ca. 25	not tested fully	ca. 10	<1
Pressor (U. per mg)	7	600	300	0—14
Antidiuretic (U. per mg)	3	600	300	32—67
Avian depressor (U. per mg)	500	85	9	<3
Oxytocic-rat uterus (U. per mg). . . .	500	30	30	0
Milk ejecting (U. per mg)	500	100		

analysis, but the similarity to vasopressin is striking. The resemblance is also seen in the pharmacological properties of CRF. Table 4 compares oxytocin, the vasopressins and CRF, and shows that, while oxytocin and vasopressin have CRF-activity at elevated doses, and vasopressin is oxytocic, CRF has some pressor and antidiuretic activity, but no oxytocic properties at the doses that were tested.

If it is possible to draw conclusions from our *in vitro* experiments, one may surmise that the neurohypophysis contains a family of chemically related peptide hormones of varying, but overlapping biological properties. While we have only tested for ACTH-releasing activity, perhaps other hypophysiotrophic hormones may be present in the hypothalamic neurohypophysial system.

Acknowledgements. Our work was made possible by generous support from a Federal Provincial Mental Health Grant (No. 604-5-425) and by a grant from the Foundations' Fund for Research in Psychiatry, both to Dr. R. A. CLEGHORN, and from N. V. ORGANON, Canada Packers Ltd., The Elizabeth Holcombe Fund of McGill University, and Charles E. Frosst and Company.

A travel grant from the Hosmer Fund of McGill University made possible attendance at the symposium.

References

1. GUILLEMIN, R., W. R. HEARN, W. R. CHEEK and D. E. HOUSHOLDER: Endocrinology **60**, 488 (1957).
2. HARRIS, G. W.: Neural Control of the Pituitary Gland. London: Edward Arnold (Publishers) Ltd. 1955.
3. SAFFRAN, M., and A. V. SCHALLY: Canad. J. Biochem. Physiol. **33**, 408 (1955).
4. — — Endocrinology **56**, 523 (1955).
5. — — and B. G. BENFEY: Endocrinology **57**, 439 (1955).
6. SCHALLY, A. V., and M. SAFFRAN: Proc. Soc. exp. Biol. (N. Y.) **92**, 636 (1956).

Istituto di Anatomia comparata dell'Università Torino, Italia

Effects of Sucrose on the Hypothalamo-hypophyseal System of Toad Tadpoles*

By

V. Mazzi and A. Guardabassi

With 2 Figures

It is known that the treatment of amphibian embryos with 10% sucrose solution produces albinism. Eakin (1953) and Driscoll and Eakin (1955) have demonstrated that the latter phenomenon depends upon the fact that the intermediate lobe fails to differentiate. This failure they regard as a consequence of

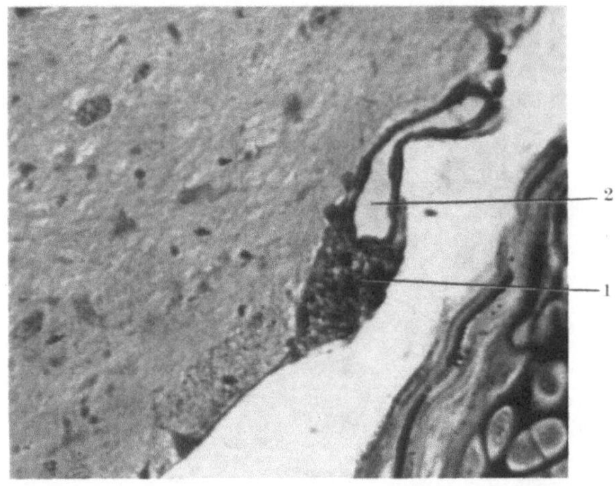

Fig. 1. 84-days larva. The praeoptico-hypophyseal tract (*1*), emerged from the brain, sticks to the internal carotid (*2*), following a forward course. Paraldehyde-fuchsin-orange; 450 ×

disturbances in gastrulation which prevent the anlage of the epithelial hypophysis from coming into contact with the infundibulum. In some cases the infundibulum does not differentiate at all. Driscoll and Eakin have shown that after treatment with sucrose the epithelial hypophysis does develop to some extent though not forming a pars intermedia; but neither of these authors nor others have been concerned with the study of the effects of these particular experimental conditions on the hypothalamo-hypophyseal system

We have studied this problem experimenting with 560 embryos of the toad, *Bufo b. bufo* (L.). Only those (160 in number) treated at the gastrula stage for as

* Research supported by a grant from C. N. R. This paper has appeared in more extensive form in Arch. Ital. Anat. Embriol. **62**, 172—196 (1957).

long as 10—14 hours have shown pigmentary effects. For histological investigations we have selected 19 albino specimens.

In two cases a normal or at least a complete if subnormal hypophysis has developed; in all the other specimens the epithelial hypophysis, though histologically differentiated, is not contiguous with the brain. The infundibulum is either poorly developed or lacking, except in two specimens in which a normal hypophysis had formed, and in two more in which the infundibulum shows a subnormal

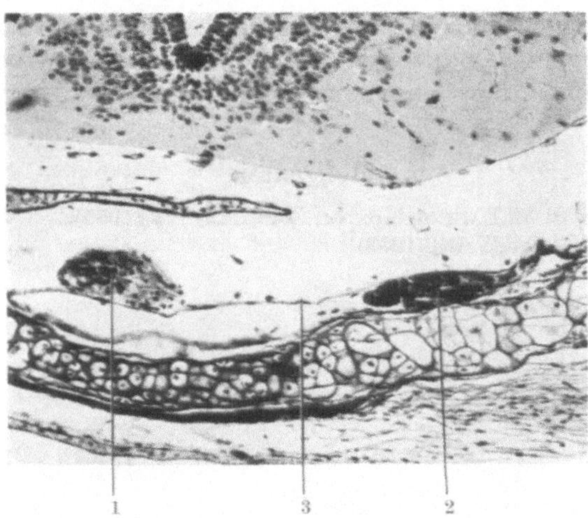

Fig. 2. 70-days larva. A subnormal infundibulum (*1*) has formed, into which the praeoptico-hypophyseal tract has penetrated. The infundibulum fails to come into contact with the adenohypophysis (*2*). The dura mater (*3*) covers the adenohypophysis and is located under the infundibulum.Paraldehyde-fuchsin-Galgano I; 100 ×

appearance. In all cases the nucleus magnocellularis praeopticus exhibits stainable neurosecretory material, even in a specimen with malformation of the praeoptic area.

The hypothalamo-hypophyseal tract has differentiated in all the larvae. It stops shortly behind the chiasma, and shows a tendency to extend beyond the brain, uni- or bilaterally, in contact with the internal carotid. In one of the two instances in which a subnormal infundibulum has developed the praeoptico-hypophyseal tract reaches the end of the infundibulum but does not form a completely differentiated neurohypophysis. The intermediate lobe fails to differentiate in these specimens, presumably because the contact between the adenohypophysis and the infundibulum is not attained, hence the disturbances in pigmentation.

The present experiments allow us to draw the following conclusions:

1) The differentiation of the nucleus magnocellularis praeopticus is independent of the presence and the extent of the territory in which its axons normally end.

2) The nucleus magnocellularis praeopticus starts its secretory activity, and the neurosecretory material flows along the fibres of the praeoptico-hypophyseal tract even though the infundibulum and the neurohypophysis are abnormal or absent.

3) In the absence of the infundibulum the praeoptico-hypophyseal tract ends shortly behind the chiasma, or else it extends beyond the brain, in contact with the internal carotid.

4) In the absence of contact between the anlage of the epithelial hypophysis and the neurohypophysis the latter is poorly developed. This is so even when a subnormal infundibulum is present into which the hypothalamo-hypophyseal tract has penetrated throughout its length.

The data resulting from our experiments and those available in the literature seem to indicate that the differentiation of the hypothalamo-hypophyseal system occurs at an early developmental stage even in the absence of normal infundibulum or contact with the adenohypophysis. Perhaps at that time they function separately, and apparently they become integrated into a harmonic system only at a later stage.

References

DRISCOLL, W. T., and R. M. EAKIN: J. exper. Zool. **129**, 149 (1955).
EAKIN, R. M.: Anat. Rec. **117**, 613 (1953).

Beobachtungen zur Morphologie der Neurosekretion bei Wirbeltieren

Von

Y. Sano (Kyoto)

Mit 9 Abbildungen, davon 2 farbige

Im folgenden werden einige Beobachtungen mitgeteilt, welche das Problem der Neurosekretion bei Wirbeltieren betreffen.

I. Lumbalmark des Rückenmarkes der Vögel

Das Lumbalmark des Rückenmarkes der Vögel enthält große multipolare Vorderhornzellen mit verschiedenen, hellen Einschlüssen im Cytoplasma, welche

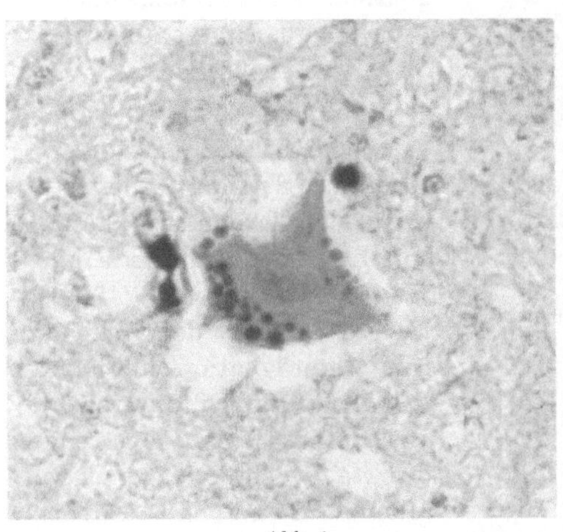

Abb. 1

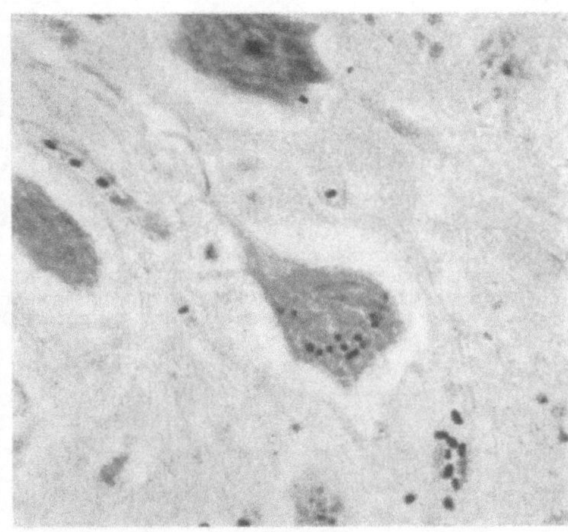

Abb. 2

Abb. 1. Mit Gentianaviolett gefärbte Einschlüsse in einer Vorderhornzelle aus dem Lumbalmark des *Haushuhns*. (Fixierung: Champysches Gemisch. Färbung: Safranin-Gentianaviolett-Orange nach FLEMMING-WINIWATER. Vergr. 520fach)

Abb. 2. Vorderhornzelle aus dem Lumbalmark des *Haushuhns*. Einschlüsse mit Eisenhämatoxylin, nach REGAUD angefärbt. (Fixierung: Zenkersches Gemisch. Färbung: Trichromfärbung nach MASSON. Vergr. 370fach)

Abb. 3. Mit Eosin gefärbte Einschlüsse in Vorderhornzellen aus dem Lumbalmark des *Haushuhns*. (Fixierung: Formol-Eisessig-Alkohol. Färbung: Methylblau-Eosin nach MANN. Vergr. 520fach)

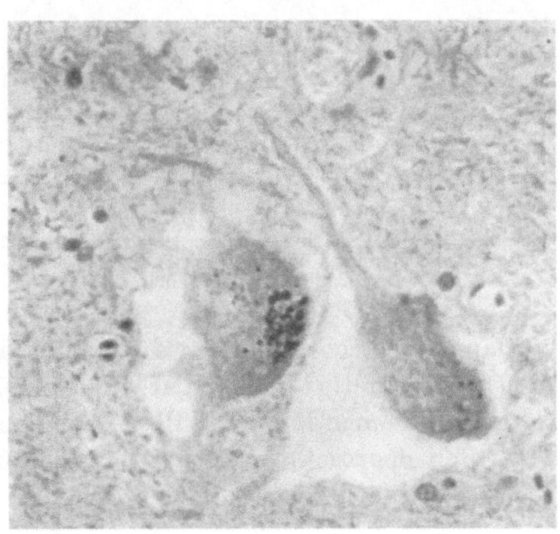

Abb. 3

siderophil, eosinophil, phloxinophil und azocarminophil sind. Für die Darstellung der Granula eignet sich besonders die Methylblau-Eosinfärbung nach Mann; sie läßt die Körnchen als leuchtend rote Gebilde hervortreten. Das Cytoplasma der einschlußhaltigen Elemente, die in allen Kerngruppen des Vorderhorns zu finden sind, zeigt keine pathologischen Veränderungen. Derartige Zellen kommen größtenteils in der Vordersäule des Lumbalmarkes, in geringer Zahl im Sacralmark vor. Wie man an mit Champy-Lösung fixierten, nach Flemming-Winiwater gefärbtem Material erkennt, sind die Einschlüsse unregelmäßig im Cytoplasma der Vorderhornzellen angeordnet, doch liegen die größeren Granula meist peripher. Einzelne große Granula werden gelegentlich auch außerhalb des Zelleibes beobachtet; offenbar werden die Einschlüsse unmittelbar in die Umgebung abgegeben. Die beschriebenen Vorderhornzellen dürften neurosekretorisch tätige Zellen sein, doch fehlt es an Hinweisen auf die chemische Natur und funktionelle Bedeutung ihrer Granula (vgl. Abb. 1—3).

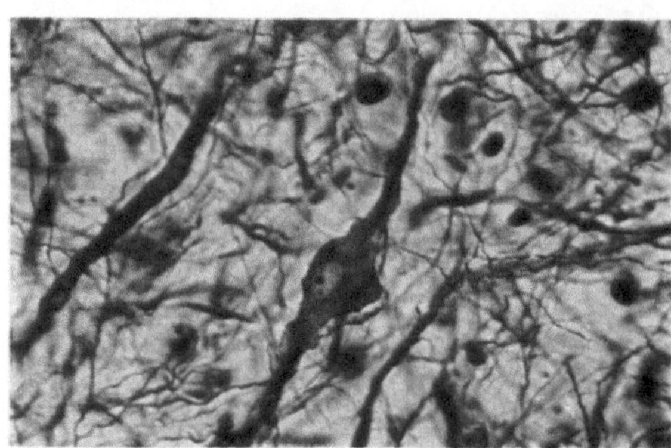

Abb. 4. Neurosekretorisch tätige Zelle im Nucleus paraventricularis vom *Hund*. (Fixierung: neutrales Formol. Färbung: Kombination der Gros-Schultzeschen Silberimprägnationsmethode mit der Aldehyd-Fuchsin-Färbung nach Gomori. Vergr. 430fach)

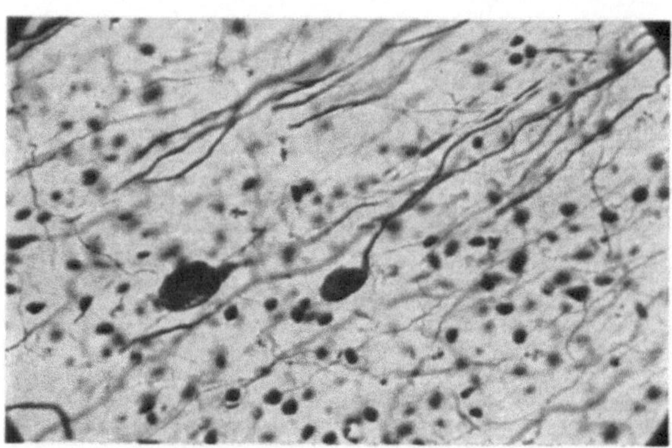

Abb. 5. Zwei mit Aldehyd-Fuchsin gefärbte Herringkörper in direkter Verbindung mit den Nervenfasern. (Technik wie bei Abb. 4. Vergr. 370fach)

II. Die Kongruenz von Imprägnations- und Färbungsbild des Tractus supraoptico-hypophyseus

Zahlreiche Autoren haben das neurosekretorische Zwischenhirn-System einerseits mit der Chromalaun-Hämatoxylin-Phloxin-Methode nach Gomori [Bargmann (1949)], andererseits mit den üblichen Silberimprägnationsmethoden für Nervenfasern untersucht. Bis heute ist jedoch der strenge direkte Nachweis der Kongruenz der mit verschiedenen Methoden darstellbaren Bahnen nicht gelungen. Deshalb habe ich versucht, diesen Nachweis mit Hilfe einer Kombination der Gros-Schultzeschen Silberimprägnationsmethode mit der Aldehyd-Fuchsin-Färbung nach Gomori zu erbringen, dabei werden die stark imprägnierten Fasern im Verlauf der Vorbereitung für die Gomori-Färbung etwas gebleicht. Wie Abb. 4, die eine neurosekretorische bipolare Zelle im Nucleus paraventricularis des Hundes wiedergibt, erkennen läßt, sind die tiefschwarz imprägnierten Fortsätze und die blaugefärbten neurosekretorischen Bahnen auf ganzer Strecke identisch (Abb. 5 u. 6).

Die Herring-Körper, bekanntlich Verdickungen von Nervenfasern, färben sich um so intensiver, je mehr ihre Argyrophilie abnimmt. Deshalb kann man in den größeren Herring-Körpern die feinen Neurofibrillenstrukturen nicht finden. Man beobachtet häufig, daß die aufgetriebenen Fasern aus zwei äußeren aldehydfuchsinophilen Zonen und aus einem inneren, nicht imprägnierten hellen Strang bestehen.

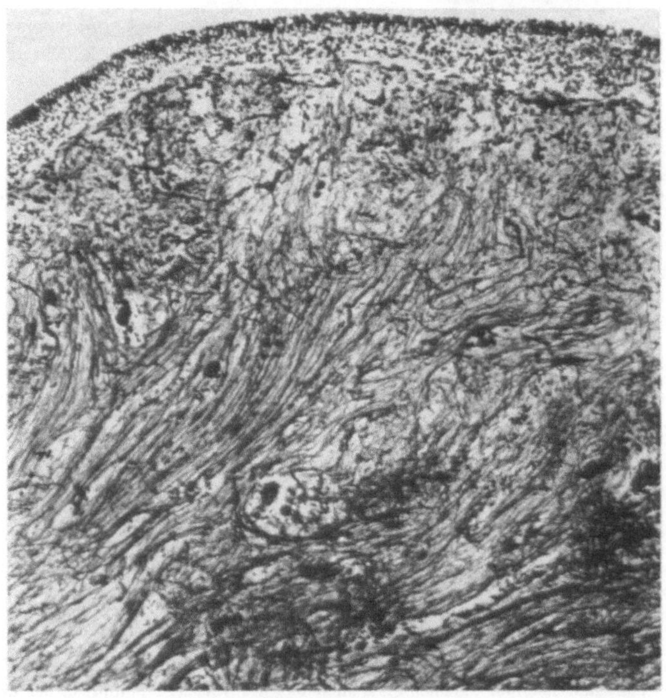

Abb. 6. Sagittalschnitt durch den Hinterlappen des *Hundes*. Nervenfasern mit Neurosekretgranula. (Technik wie bei Abb. 4. Vergr. 96fach)

III. Neuroglia im Nucleus supraopticus und paraventricularis

Für die Darstellung der Neurogliazellen im Hypothalamus-Hypophysen-system von Hund und Katze erwies sich die YANOsche Warmformalinmethode (1952, 1953) als die geeignetste. Die Neurogliazellen im Gebiet des Nucleus supraopticus sind untereinander durch Fortsätze netzartig verbunden; eine Anzahl dieser Fortsätze endet mit Gliafüßchen an der Oberfläche der neurosekretorischen Zellen. Häufig ließen sich Verbindungen der Neurogliazellen mit den Capillaren und neurosekretorischen Zellen in Gestalt von Fortsätzen nachweisen. Bei Hund und Katze konnten die bekannten Neurogliazelltypen im Bereich des Nucleus supraopticus nicht dargestellt werden. Welche spezifische Bedeutung die hier beschriebenen Neurogliazellen für die Funktion des Kerngebietes haben, ist eine offene Frage. Man kann lediglich vermuten, daß die neurosekretorischen Zellen durch ihre Vermittlung mit den zahlreichen Capillargefäßen in Stoffaustausch stehen (Abb. 7 u. 8).

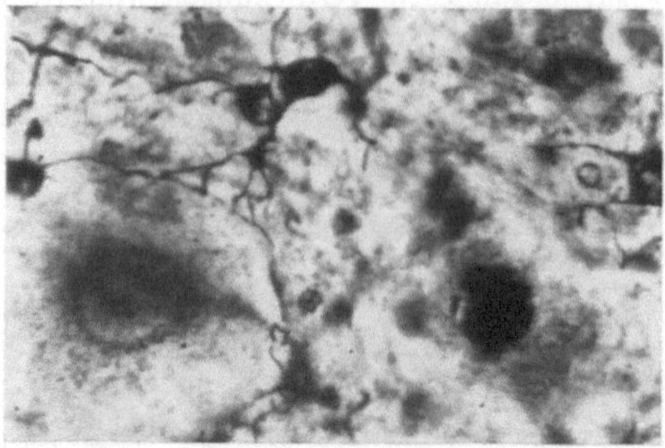

Abb. 7. Neurogliazellen im Gebiet des Nucleus paraventricularis der *Katze*, die mit Gliafüßchen an die Oberfläche der neurosekretorischen Zellen herantreten. (Fixierung: neutrales Formol. Gefrierschnitt. Yanosche Warmformolmethode. Vergr. 430fach)

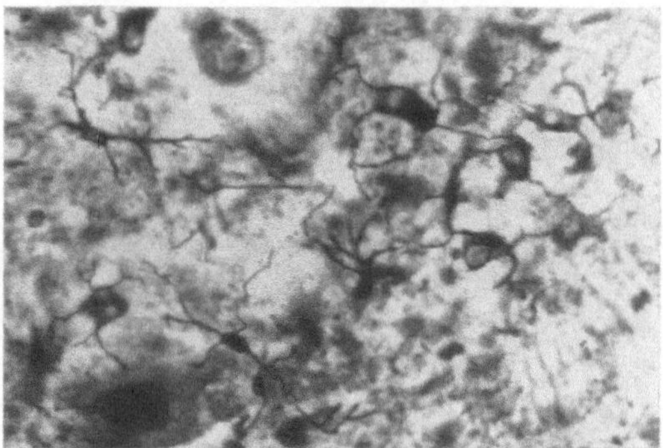

Abb. 8. Neurogliazellen und Ganglienzellen im Gebiet des Nucleus supraopticus der *Katze*. (Technik wie bei Abb. 7. Vergr. 430fach)

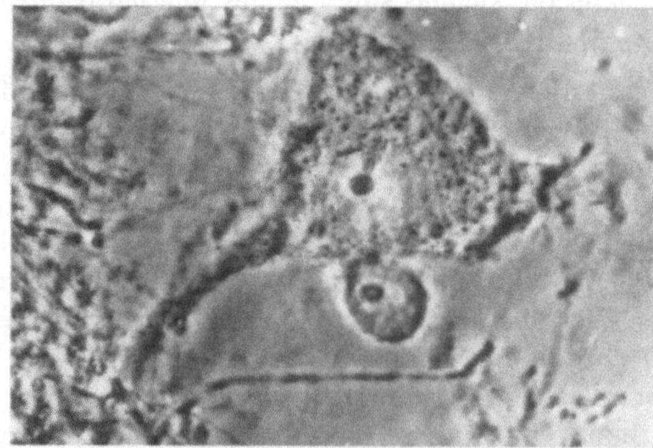

Abb. 9. Ganglienzelle mit Neurosekretgranula im Nucleus supraopticus des *Hundes*. (Frisches unfixiertes Material. Zupfpräparat. Phasenkontrast-Mikrophotographie, PM. Vergr. 650fach)

IV. Neurosekret

1. Nachweis von Neurosekret im Nucleus supraopticus des normalen und durstenden Hundes mit dem Phasenkontrastverfahren. In den Nervenzellen des Nucleus supraopticus vom Hunde kann man mit Hilfe des Phasenkontrastverfahrens dunkle kleine Granula zwischen der Nissl-Substanz nachweisen. Diese Granula sind beim durstenden Versuchstier weitgehend aus dem Cytoplasma der Ganglienzellen verschwunden. Sie treten wiederum in Erscheinung, wenn sich der Hund durch Wasseraufnahme erholt hat. Gleichartige Granula gibt es in den Pyramidenzellen oder in den Purkinje-Zellen nicht. Deshalb darf man annehmen, daß diese Granula Neurosekret darstellen und auch im frischen, unfixierten Objekt in granulärer Form vorliegen. Die sog. "linear striation" PALAYs (1953) wurde vermißt (Abb. 9).

2. Elektronenoptische Darstellung des Neurosekrets. Im elektronenmikroskopischen Bild läßt sich im Einklang mit PALAY (1955, 1957), FUJITA (1957), BARGMANN und KNOOP (1957) und anderen Untersuchern zeigen, daß im Cytoplasma der marklosen Fasern des Tractus supraoptico-hypophyseus vom Hunde charakteristische Elementargranula enthalten sind. An diesen Granula läßt sich ein massendichterer Kern ausmachen, der von einer Membran umschlossen ist. Zwischen letzterer und dem Internum befindet sich eine schmale, hellere Randzone. An welchen Anteil des Elementarkörnchens die Hinterlappenhormone gebunden sind, ist unbekannt.

Literatur

BARGMANN, W., u. A. KNOOP: Z. Zellforsch. **46**, 242—251 (1957).
FUJITA, H.: Arch. Histol. jap. **12**, 165—172 (1957).
PALAY, S. L.: Anat. Rec. **121**, 348 (1957).
— Progr. in Neurobiology, Vol. II. New York: P. B. Hoeber 1957.
YANO, K.: Folia Psychiat. Neurol. jap. **5**, 181 (1952).
— Psychiat. Neurol. jap. **55**, 528 (1953).

Fysiologiska Institutionen, Karolinska Institutet, Stockholm, Sweden

Occurrence of Substance P in the Central Nervous System of Fish

By

U. S. VON EULER and E. ÖSTLUND

In 1931 EULER and GADDUM observed that extracts of mammalian intestine and brain contained a substance which stimulated intestinal motility. The active principle which exerts its action also in the presence of atropine can be extracted from intestine and brain by boiling at p_H 4 and subsequent precipitation with ammonium sulphate [EULER (1936a)]. The activity disappears after incubation with trypsin [EULER (1936b)]. The active substance, which was provisionally named Substance P, is stable at boiling temperature at p_H 4 [GADDUM and SCHILD (1934)] and is dialysable. It shows the general properties of a polypeptide.

A relatively simple and efficient method for its purification was elaborated in 1953 by PERNOW who showed that it was quantitatively adsorbed on aluminium oxide from a 70% solution in methanol or ethanol. By elution with falling concentrations of the solvent most of the activity was recovered in a highly purified form in a few fractions.

Further purification was obtained by partition chromatography on a cellulose column or paper, the maximal activity corresponding to about 3 units per μg. The biological standard unit causes a well marked increase in the tone and amplitude of the isolated rabbit's jejunum in a 30 ml bath. It was shown by PERNOW (1955) that the activity was readily destroyed by small concentrations of chymotrypsin, further supporting the assumption that the substance was of polypeptide nature. A comparative study between the active substances prepared in the same way from intestine and brain, using chromatography, counter current distribution and inactivation tests, showed that the preparations were identical [ELIASSON, LIE and PERNOW (1956)].

Table 1. *Distribution of Substance P in the Nervous System (dog)* (PERNOW, 1953)

Medulla spinalis . .	35 units/g
Cerebellum	15
Hypothalamus . . .	170
Basal ganglia . . .	150
Spinal nerve	20
Phrenic nerve . . .	7

The distribution of Substance P in the different layers of the small intestine and in the various parts of the central and peripheral nervous systems has been studied by a number of authors [for ref. see PERNOW (1955), and PAASONEN and VOGT (1956)]. The concentration was remarkably high in some parts of the brain, especially the hypothalamus, which contained 170 U. per g in the dog (Table 1). In general the activity was considerably higher in the gray than in the white matter. The accumulation of Substance P in some portions of the brain suggests that it may be of functional importance in these parts. LEMBECK (1953) found large amounts of Substance P in the dorsal roots and suggested a relationship between Substance P and the sensory nerve transmittor.

Central effects of Substance P were studied by EULER and PERNOW (1956) who administered the substance intracisternally and intraventricularly in rabbits and cats. The injections elicited an increase in respiration but mostly only slight changes in the blood pressure. In other experiments changes in the mood of the animals were observed. Licking movements and salivation were not infrequent.

In a study on the effects of Substance P on mice ZETLER (1956) has described a number of actions on the central nervous system, such as sedating action, a potentiation of barbiturate action, hyperalgesia, and an antagonistic action towards morphia.

Since Substance P is regularly found in the intestine and brain of mammals, including man, it seemed of interest to examine its occurrence also in other animal classes and phyla. The present report deals with its occurrence in the central nervous system of various classes of fish including the hagfish.

Extracts were prepared from the brain of the freshly caught hagfish *(Myxine glutinosa)* and the codfish *(Gadus callarias)* and the brain and spinal cord of a ray *(Raja batis)*. The organs were minced, boiled for 5 min. in 2 volumes of water at p_H 4, and the filtrate saturated to 70% with ammonium sulphate. The precipitate was dissolved in water, and methanol added slowly to 70%. The voluminous precipitate was discarded and the clear solution passed through an aluminium oxide column and eluted with falling concentrations of methanol. The activity of the separate fractions, freed from methanol, was assayed against a standard on the isolated guinea-pig's ileum in the presence of atropine and antasten. Active samples were routinely incubated with trypsine, which completely inactivated them in the same way as the standard. The extracts were also assayed on the isolated rabbit's intestine, and the blood pressure of the cat and the rabbit.

The results are given in Table 2.

Table 2. *Substance P in Brain and Spinal Cord of Fish*

Species	Number of animals	Organ	Total weight of organ g	Activity units "P" per g
Hagfish (Myxine glutinosa) .	173	Whole brain	3.0	3.3
Codfish (Gadus callarias) . .	13	Whole brain	15.3	6.0
Ray (Raia batis)	7	Olfactory brain	11.5	5.1
Ray (Raia batis)	7	Rest of brain	23.5	8.5
Ray (Raia batis)	6	Spinal cord	11	19
Ray (Raia batis)	7	Spinal cord	29	36

From this study it emerges that Substance P is present in the brain of teleosts *(Gadus callarias)* as well as in that of elasmobranchs *(Raja batis)* and of cyclostomes *(Myxine glutinosa)*. While the amounts of Substance P in the intestine of the hagfish were much less than in the intestine of both *Gadus* and *Raja*, the content in the brain was comparable to that in the other species. In the ray the olfactory brain contained less than the rest of the brain. Particularly high amounts were found in the spinal cord of the ray, which contained up to 36 units per g.

Summary

Substance P, a polypeptide which is present in mammalian intestine and brain and stimulates the smooth muscle of the intestine and exerts certain actions on the central nervous system, is present in the brain of the codfish *(Gadus callarias)*, the ray *(Raja batis)* and the hagfish *(Myxine glutinosa)* in amounts of 3.3—8.5 units per g. Large amounts were found in the spinal cord of *Raja batis* (19—36 units per g).

The high concentration of substance P in the mammalian hypothalamus might suggest that the hypothalamic neurosecretory cells produce this polypeptide in addition to those known to be elaborated by them, namely vasopressin and oxytocin. However, the latter are found only in areas of neurosecretory cells, whereas substance P occurs in parts other than the hypothalamus although in lower concentrations. Substance P may be classified as a neurohumor, not as a neurohormone. It appears that it is produced by a variety of cells, not necessarily by neurosecretory cells.

References

Eliasson, R., L. Lie and B. Pernow: Brit. J. Pharmacol. **11**, 137 (1956).
Euler, U. S. v.: Naunyn-Schmiedebergs Arch. exp. Path. Pharmak. **181**, 181 (1936a).
— Skand. Arch. Physiol. **73**, 142 (1936b).
— and J. H. Gaddum: J. Physiol. **72**, 74 (1931).
— and B. Pernow: Acta physiol. scand. **36**, 265 (1956).
Gaddum, J. H., and H. Schild: J. Physiol. **83**, 1 (1934).
Lembeck, F.: Naunyn-Schmiedebergs Arch. exp. Path. Pharmak. **219**, 197 (1953).
Paasonen, M. K., and M. Vogt: J. Physiol. **131**, 617 (1956).
Pernow, B.: Acta physiol. scand. **29**, Suppl. 105 (1953).
— Acta physiol. scand. **34**, 295 (1955).
— Z. Vitamin-, Hormon- u. Fermentforsch. **7**, 59 (1955).
Zetler, G.: Naunyn-Schmiedebergs Arch. exp. Path. Pharmak. **228**, 513 (1956).

Laboratoire de Chimie Biologique de la Faculté des Sciences de Marseille, France

Etat naturel des principes ocytocique et vasopressique de la neurohypophyse

Par

ROGER ACHER

Avec 2 Figures

L'isolement d'une substance active à partir d'un extrait de glande pose deux questions importantes: 1°) la substance isolée existe-t-elle à l'état naturel dans l'organe, c'est-à-dire représente-t-elle le principe actif physiologique et non un produit artificiellement modifié au cours de l'extraction ? 2°) L'existence à l'état naturel de la substance étant admise, quelle est sa signification biochimique c'est-à-dire s'agit-il d'une forme de synthèse, de réserve, ou de sécrétion du principe actif ? En effet, alors que bien souvent on suppose qu'à une activité spécifique correspond une substance chimique unique, en réalité la forme chimique sous laquelle un principe actif est synthétisé par l'organisme n'est pas obligatoirement celle sous laquelle le principe est mis en réserve, ni celle sous laquelle le principe est sécrété. Le cas des hormones thyroïdiennes est caractéristique à cet égard. On peut donc envisager l'existence de plusieurs substances chimiques, toutes douées de l'activité spécifique et représentant normalement différentes étapes de transformation de l'hormone entre la synthèse et la sécrétion.

Dans le cas du complexe hypothalamo-hypophysaire, on admet généralement à la suite de BARGMANN et SCHARRER (3) que les principes ocytocique et vasopressique sont synthétisés au niveau des noyaux supraoptiques et paraventriculaires de l'hypothalamus, puis sont transportés le long des axones de la tige pituitaire jusqu'au lobe postérieur de l'hypophyse où ils s'accumulent et d'où ils seront secrétés. Si la présence des activités ocytocique et vasopressique au niveau des noyaux hypothalamiques, de la tige et de la post-hypophyse peut servir d'argument en faveur de cette conception, elle n'indique nullement que la substance chimique à activité ocytocique, par exemple, est la même dans l'hypothalamus, la tige et la post-hypophyse. Les substances actives de l'hypothalamus (forme de synthèse) ainsi que celles du sang (forme de sécrétion) n'ont pas été obtenues à l'état suffisamment pures pour être caractérisées chimiquement. Jusqu'à présent, seules ont été effectivement isolées, les substances actives se trouvant dans le lobe postérieur de l'hypophyse de boeuf et de porc.

Ces substances sont au nombre de 3: 1° La protéine de VAN DYKE (21), protéine d'un poids moléculaire d'environ 30000, qui possède les quatre activités ocytocique, galactagogue, vasopressique et antidiurétique dans le rapport où ces activités existent dans la glande c'est-à-dire 1:1. 2° L'ocytocine (12, 13), peptide d'un poids moléculaire de 1000 environ possédant principalement les activités ocytocique et galactagogue. 3° La vasopressine (7, 19), peptide ayant approximativement le même poids moléculaire que l'ocytocine et possédant principalement les activités vasopressique et antidiurétique.

Etat naturel des principes actifs de la post-hypophyse

La première question à résoudre était de déterminer si ces trois substances existent bien à l'état naturel dans la glande. VAN DYKE et ses collaborateurs (21) d'une dart ayant isolé la protéine active dans des conditions très douces (extraction à froid, précipitation par le chlorure de sodium, dialyse) d'autre part ayant contrôlé sa pureté par des expériences d'ultracentrifugation, d'électrophorèse et par le test de solubilité, ont considéré la protéine active comme l'hormone véritable. Les peptides ocytocine et vasopressine sont isolés dans des conditions plus brutales (notamment extraction à chaud par l'acide acétique dilué). Ils pourraient être obtenus par dégradation de la «molécule-mère». Sur la base de ces données, on envisageait deux possibilités: 1° La protéine active est l'hormone véritable et les peptides ocytocine et vasopressine ne sont que des fragments encore actifs formés au cours de l'extraction. 2° La protéine active est un précurseur commun à l'ocytocine et à la vasopressine. Dans ce cas les trois substances existent à l'état naturel dans la glande, la protéine étant une forme de réserve et les peptides étant des formes de sécrétion. Cependant avant d'avancer une interprétation quelconque, il était nécessaire de vérifier soigneusement que les activités biologiques appartiennent d'une façon intrinsèque aux produits considérés et non à des impuretés présentes à l'état de trace. S'il ne fait aucun doute que les peptides ocytocine et vasopressine possèdent en propre respectivement l'activité ocytocique et l'activité vasopressique, il n'en est pas de même pour la protéine. Il nous a paru important de contrôler son homogénéité par différentes méthodes et d'observer si au cours de divers traitements ne produisant aucune dégradation, les activités biologiques restaient toujours associées à la protéine.

Nous avons préparé la protéine active à partir de post-hypophyses de boeuf dans les conditions décrites par VAN DYKE et al. (21). Le poids moléculaire déterminé d'après la constante de sédimentation et la constante de diffusion est 30.000 environ. La teneur en azote est de 15,9%. La protéine ne contient pas de sucres. Elle est très riche en cystine et en proline. Elle est peu soluble dans l'eau pure mais soluble dans l'acide acétique dilué ou l'ammoniaque dilué. Au point de vue biologique, la protéine présente une activité ocytocique et une activité vasopressique de 18—20 u.i./mg.

Nous avons soumis la protéine à divers traitements ne mettant en jeu aucune hydrolyse, de façon à vérifier sa pureté.

1° *Electrodialyse*. 50 mg de protéine active dissous dans 35 ml d'eau à l'aide d'une trace d'acide acétique sont placés dans le compartiment central d'un électrodialyseur à 3 compartiments. Les compartiments anodique et cathodique contiennent de l'eau et les membranes sont de cellophane. La protéine ne peut passer la membrane de cellophane. On applique une tension d'environ 1000 volts pendant une dizaine d'heures. On observe alors que 90 à 100% des activités ont passé la membrane et se trouvent dans le compartiment cathodique alors que la protéine est restée dans le compartiment central. L'étude des produits du compartiment cathodique par électrophorèse sur papier permet d'identifier l'ocytocine et la vasopressine qui seules sont responsables des activités. La protéine active apparaît donc en réalité comme une association entre une protéine dépourvue d'activité et les deux peptides ocytocine et vasopressine responsables des activités.

2° *Précipitation par l'acide trichloracétique.* L'acide trichloracétique précipite les protéines mais laisse les peptides en solution. C'est un agent utilisé pour séparer les protéines des peptides. La protéine active en solution à 1% est précipitée par l'acide trichloracétique à 5%. Le liquide surnageant renferme 50 à 70% des activités. L'étude par électrophorèse sur papier des produits actifs du liquide surnageant permet d'identifier l'ocytocine et la vasopressine. On identifie également les deux peptides par chromatographie du liquide surnageant sur colonne de résine échangeur d'ions: l'Amberlite IRC 50 (Fig. 1).

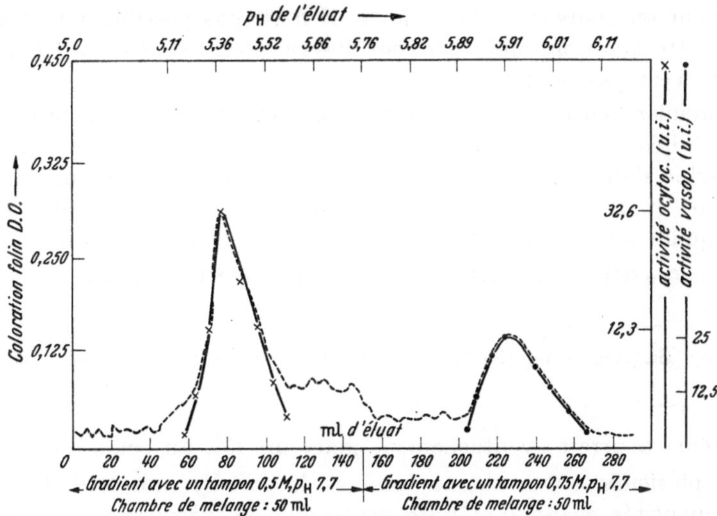

Fig. 1. Chromatographie sur Amberlite IRC 50 (XE 64) des peptidenson precipites par l'acide trichloracétique. (Colonne 0.9 × 10 cm. initialement équilibrée avec un tampon acétate NH₄ 0.1 M, pH 5)

L'acide trichloracétique dissocie donc la protéine active en une protéine inerte d'une part, l'ocytocine et la vasopressine d'autre part.

3° *Distribution à contre-courant.* La protéine (20 mg) est soumise à la distribution par contre-courant dans le système butanol secondaire-acide trichloracétique 0,5%. Après 24 transferts, on dose dans les tubes les activités et l'azote. On constate alors que la substance à activité vasopressique se trouve dans les tubes 8 à 10, la substance à activité ocytocique dans les tubes 11 à 15 et la protéine sans activité dans les tubes 15 à 21. Les substances actives sont isolées et on peut identifier par chromatographie sur papier respectivement l'ocytocine et la vasopressine. La distribution à contre-courant a donc dissocié la protéine active en une protéine inerte d'une part, l'ocytocine et la vasopressine d'autre part.

Donc trois procédés: l'électrodialyse, la précipitation par l'acide trichloracétique, la distribution à contre-courant, indiquent que la protéine active n'est pas une protéine pure mais est en réalité une association entre une protéine dépourvue d'activité, que nous proposons d'appeler *neurophysine,* et deux peptides actifs l'*ocytocine* et la *vasopressine*. En conséquence les résultats obtenus conduisent aux conclusions suivantes:

1° L'ocytocine et la vasopressine existent à l'état naturel dans la glande puisqu'on peut les isoler après une extraction à froid et dans des conditions très douces.

2° L'ocytocine et la vasopressine sont les seules substances possédant respectivement les activités ocytocique et vasopressique qui existent dans la post-hypophyse. Il n'existe pas une protéine pure douée à la fois des deux activités.

Signification biologique de l'association protéine-peptides

La question qui se pose immédiatement est la suivante: l'association protéine-peptides possède-t-elle une signification biologique ou bien est-elle réalisée artificiellement au cours de l'extraction? Il n'est pas possible actuellement de répondre à cette question, mais certaines observations sembleraient indiquer que l'association n'est pas un fait du hasard.

1° En premier lieu l'association semble se faire molécule à molécule. Sur la base des activités, on peut calculer qu'une molécule d'ocytocine et une molécule de vasopressine s'unissent à une molécule de protéine. Les structures chimiques de l'ocytocine et de la vasopressine de boeuf sont très voisines et il n'est pas impossible qu'un certain stade de la biosynthèse soit commun aux deux peptides.

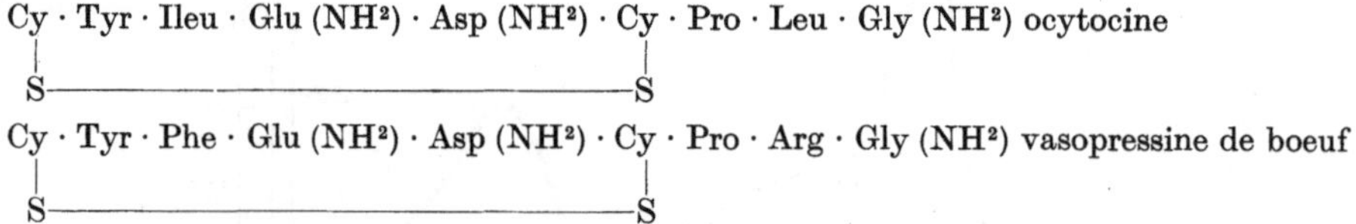

La protéine pourrait éventuellement jouer un rôle au cours de la synthèse.

2° Chez plusieurs espèces de mammifères, la post-hypophyse de l'adulte contient des quantités égales d'activité ocytocique et vasopressique. Ceci a été constaté chez l'homme, le rat, le chat, le chien, le mouton, le porc et le cheval (9, 16, 23, 5, 6). La présence des deux activités dans un rapport 1:1 peut suggérer l'existence chez ces espèces d'une association identique à celle qui a été mise en évidence chez le boeuf. Nous avons cherché à vérifier cette hypothèse. A partir de glandes de porc, nous avons pu préparer un produit qui paraît très semblable à celui isolé des glandes de boeuf. La teneur en azote, les constantes de sédimentation et de diffusion sont pratiquement identiques. Le produit possède les deux activités ocytocique et vasopressique dans un rapport 1:1, ces activités étant comme dans le cas du produit d'origine bovine, de 18 u.i./mg. On peut également effectuer la dissociation entre une protéine inerte et les deux peptides actifs par électrodialyse, par précipitation au moyen de l'acide trichloracétique et par distribution à contre-courant. Des recherches sont en cours pour établir si l'association existe chez d'autres espèces.

Cependant DICKER et TYLER (5, 6) ont noté que chez le jeune, l'activité vasopressique est supérieure à l'activité ocytocique. Nous avons étudié la variation du rapport activité vasopressique/activité ocytocique dans la neurohypophyse du rat au cours de la croissance: ce rapport, qui est de 12 chez l'animal de 5 jours, diminue progressivement pour devenir égal à 1 chez l'animal de 40 jours. Doit-on conclure que l'association est formée tardivement dans la neurohypophyse, vers le 40ème jour, ou bien qu'elle existe bien avant mais que l'ocytocine est présente dans cette association sous une forme encore inactive, une «pro-hormone»? Ces observations sont à rapprocher de celles de Vogt (22) qui a constaté que le rapport activité vasopressique/activité ocytocique est de 14 dans l'hypothalamus de chien, alors que ce même rapport est de 1 dans la neurohypophyse. Envisageant plusieurs explications, l'auteur estime qu'une modification pourrait s'effectuer pendant le transport de la ou des substances de l'hypothalamus à la neurohypophyse, modification qui ferait apparaître l'activité ocytocique.

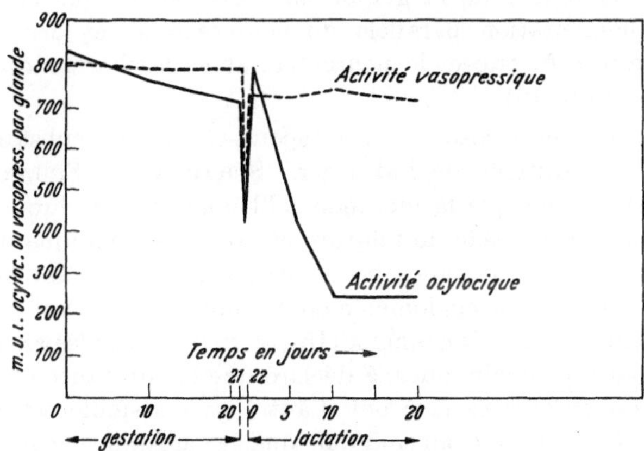

Fig. 2. Variations des activités ocytocique et vasopressique dans la neurohypophyse
de la rate au cours de la reproduction

Les informations sur la biosynthèse des hormones sont encore trop peu nombreuses pour permettre d'avoir une conception, même très générale, de son mécanisme. Toutefois il est possible que l'association soit un des stades de ce mécanisme.

3° Quel est le destin de l'association au moment de la sécrétion des hormones? Se comporte-t-elle comme un tout, c'est-à-dire la protéine et les deux peptides sont-ils sécrétés ensemble? Un certain nombre d'observations ont été faites qui plaident en faveur d'une sécrétion simultanée des deux principes actifs [cf. Revues de van Dyke (20) et de Heller (8)]. Nous avons étudié les variations des activités vasopressique et ocytocique dans la neurohypophyse du rat au cours de la gestation, de la parturition et de la lactation (Fig. 2). Chez l'animal normal les quantités des deux activités sont sensiblement égales et voisines de 800 mu par glande. Au cours de la gestation on n'observe pas de variation significative. Au moment de la parturition, 50% des deux activités sont sécrétées, ce qui pourrait être interprété comme une sécrétion du complexe protéine-ocytocine-vasopressine. Si on laisse les petits têter, il y a, après 24 heures, reconstitution simultanée des quantités initiales d'hormones. Pendant la lactation seule l'activité ocytocique est sécrétée: dans ces conditions il y a dissociation du complexe. En conséquence si dans certains cas l'association pourrait être sécrétée comme un tout (parturition), dans d'autres, comme au cours de la lactation, la sécrétion isolée d'une seule hormone est possible.

4° Des observations cytologiques, en particulier l'examen de coupes colorées à l'aide de la technique de GOMORI-BARGMANN (2), ont mis en évidence dans le système hypothalamo-neurohypophysaire un matériel de neurosécrétion. Cette substance dite «Gomori-positive» a suscité un grand intérêt parce qu'elle semblait avoir un destin parallèle à celui des hormones neurohypophysaires. Quelles sont les relations qui existent entre la substance «Gomori-positive» et l'association que nous venons d'étudier?

On a observé très souvent que la diminution de la substance «Gomori-positive» dans la neurohypophyse obtenue par deshydratation des animaux coïncide avec la diminution de la teneur de la glande en hormones et que la réhydratation détermine une augmentation parallèle du neurosécrétat et des hormones (8). Si la tige pituitaire est coupée, le neurosécrétat et les hormones s'accumulent au-dessus de la section (10).

La substance «Gomori-positive» correspond-elle à une substance chimique bien définie? Il est difficile de l'affirmer. SCHARRER et SCHARRER (14) ont souligné avec juste raison que la méthode à l'hématoxyline chromique-phloxine de GOMORI n'est qu'un procédé de teinture et non une technique histochimique. Il faut remarquer que la substance ne devient perceptible avec la méthode de coloration que lorsqu'elle est agglomérée en granules, renfermant chacun un très grand nombre de molécules. SCHIEBLER (15), se fondant sur les résultats obtenus à l'aide de méthodes histochimiques, a déclaré que la substance était une gluco-lipoprotéine. HILD et ZETLER (11) ont d'autre part assimilé cette substance à un phosphatide. Ces auteurs ont indiqué que la substance «Gomori-positive» pouvait être extraite de la neurohypophyse par un mélange alcool-chloroforme alors que les hormones restaient à l'intérieur de la glande. Ils ont conclu que la substance Gomori-positive n'est pas responsable des activités.

Nous avons effectué la réaction de GOMORI sur l'association active en déposant sur lames de verre environ 100 μg de produit et en effectuant le traitement classique (2). L'association active donne la coloration. Lorsque cette association est dissociée, soit par électrodialyse, soit par distribution à contre-courant la protéine *neurophysine* donne la coloration, mais les peptides *ocytocine* et *vaso-pressine* ne la donnent pas. Cette observation rejoint celle de HILD et ZETLER suivant laquelle les hormones ne sont pas les substances colorables par la réaction de GOMORI. Il est prématuré d'affirmer que la protéine représente la substance «Gomori-positive» des cellules en se fondant sur le simple fait d'une identité de coloration. Toutefois certaines observations récentes seraient en faveur de cette conception. SLOPER (17, 1) a repris les investigations sur la nature chimique de la substance «Gomori-positive» à l'aide de techniques histochimiques nouvelles. Il montre que la substance n'est pas soluble dans les solvants organiques et qu'elle ne contient ni sucres ni lipides. En utilisant diverses réactions spécifiques des ponts disulfures, il met en évidence sa richesse en cystine. D'après les résultats obtenus, la substance «Gomori-positive» n'est ni une glucolipoprotéine, ni un phosphatide mais un peptide ou une protéine riche en cystine.

De même BARRNETT (4) observe la présence de ponts disulfures dans la substance. Sur la base de ces données la protéine neurophysine, qui ne contient ni sucres ni lipides mais qui est riche en cystine, pourrait être la substance

«Gomori-positive». Des preuves supplémentaires sont nécessaires avant d'admettre cette hypothèse. Il est intéressant de noter que les comportements de la substance «Gomori-positive» et des hormones, quoique souvent parallèles, sont quelquefois différents. STUTINSKY (18) a noté chez le rat que la parturition ne s'accompagnait pas d'une diminution de la substance «GOMORI» de la neurohypophyse. La diminution n'a lieu que si on laisse les petits têter c'est-à-dire la lactation se produire. Nous avons constaté que la parturition s'accompagne d'une baisse de 50% des activités vasopressique et ocytocique. Si on laisse les petits têter, il y a au contraire augmentation de la teneur en hormones qui devient normale en quelques heures. Si on ne laisse pas les petits têter, l'augmentation est très lente. Il semble dans ce cas particulier que la disparition de la substance «Gomori» s'accompagne d'une apparition des principes actifs.

En conclusion il apparaît que: 1° La substance «Gomori-positive» ne représente pas les hormones. Son rôle dans la biosynthèse, le transport ou l'activation des hormones demeure jusqu'à présent entièrement hypothétique.

2° La substance «Gomori-positive» pourrait être soit la protéine *neurophysine* qui participe à une association particulière protéine-ocytocine-vasopressine, soit une substance chimiquement voisine. Mais la réaction de GOMORI n'est pas assez spécifique pour justifier l'identification.

Résumé

L'étude des substances de la neurohypophyse, douées des activités ocytocique et vasopressique a conduit aux conclusions suivantes:

1° Les peptides *ocytocine* et *vasopressine* existent à l'état naturel dans la glande et doivent être considérés comme de véritables substances physiologiques.

2° La neurohypophyse ne contient pas une protéine pure douée à la fois des activités ocytocique et vasopressique qui pourrait être considérée comme un précurseur commun de l'*ocytocine* et de la *vasopressine*, ou comme une forme de réserve des hormones. Cependant l'*ocytocine* et la *vasopressine* semblent associées, au moins chez certaines espèces, à une protéine dépourvue d'activité, la *neurophysine*.

3° La signification biologique de l'association *neurophysine-ocytocine-vasopressine* demeure hypothétique. La *neurophysine* pourrait être le matériel colorable au sein des cellules par la réaction de GOMORI-BARGMANN mais cette réaction n'est pas assez spécifique pour justifier l'identification.

Bibliographie

1. ADAMS, C. W. M., and J. C. SLOPER: J. Endocr. **13**, 221 (1956).
2. BARGMANN, W.: Z. Zellforsch. **34**, 610 (1949).
3. — and E. SCHARRER: Amer. Scientist **39**, 255 (1951).
4. BARRNETT, R. J.: Endocrinology **55**, 484 (1954).
5. DICKER, S. E., and C. TYLER: J. Physiol. **120**, 141 (1953).
6. — — J. Physiol. **121**, 206 (1953).
7. FROMAGEOT, P., R. ACHER, H. CLAUSER and M. MAIER-HÜSER: Biochim. biophys. Acta **12**, 424 (1953).
8. HELLER, H.: J. Pharm. (Lond.) **7**, 225 (1955).
9. — and E. J. ZAIMIS: J. Physiol. **109**, 162 (1949).

10. HILD, W., u. G. ZETLER: Pflüg. Arch. ges. Physiol. **257**, 169 (1953).
11. — — Z. ges. exp. Med. **120**, 236 (1953).
12. MAIER-HÜSER, H., H. CLAUSER, P. FROMAGEOT et R. PLONGERON: Biochim. biophys. Acta **11**, 252 (1953).
13. PIERCE, J. G., and V. DU VIGNEAUD: J. biol. Chem. **186**, 77 (1950).
14. SCHARRER, E., and B. SCHARRER: Recent Progr. Hormone Res. **10**, 183 (1954).
15. SCHIEBLER, T. H.: Z. Zellforsch. **36**, 563 (1952).
16. SIMON, A.: Amer. J. Physiol. **107**, 220 (1934).
17. SLOPER, J. C.: J. Anat. **88**, 576 (1954).
18. STUTINSKY, F.: Ann. d'Endocr. **14**, 722 (1953).
19. TURNER, R. A., J. G. PIERCE and V. DU VIGNEAUD: J. biol. Chem. **191**, 21 (1951).
20. VAN DYKE, H. B., K. ADAMSONS and S. L. ENGEL: Recent Progr. Hormone Res. **11**, 1 (1955).
21. VAN DYKE, H. B., B. F. CHOW, R. O. GREEP, and A. ROTHEN: J. Pharmacol. Exptl. Therap. **74**, 190 (1942).
22. VOGT, M.: Brit. J. Pharmacol. **8**, 193 (1953).
23. WARING, H., and F. W. LANDGREBE: In G. PINCUS and K. V. THIMAN, The Hormones. Vol. 2, p. 427. New York: Academic Press Inc. 1950.

Department of Anatomy, Albert Einstein College of Medicine, New York

Neuro-endocrine Mechanisms in Insects*

By

BERTA SCHARRER

With 2 Figures

One of the more important questions upon which present interest in endo-crinology is focused concerns those factors which control the activities of the glands of internal secretion. What are these factors, and in which way is their influence transmitted to the endocrine organs so as to result in integrated action ? Known factors of this kind are either external, such as light, temperature, and humidity, or internal, such as a given metabolic condition or the functional state of a specific effector organ.

As to the manner in which these factors influence the activity of the endocrine organs, it has become increasingly clear that they frequently do not seem to act on the target glands directly but by way of one or more intermediary mechanisms, one of which is in the central nervous system. In other words, there exist chain reactions in which nervous and endocrine steps may alternate with each other. The routing of stimuli from the external and internal milieu through the central nervous system makes possible the analysis and integration of diverse influences before a definitive message is sent to the target gland. The nervous system is ideally suited to serve as such a way-station, since it is capable of both receiving and dispatching nervous as well as hormonal messages.

An endocrine gland, provided it possesses the appropriate nerve supply, may be activated or restrained by nervous action. Where this nervous pathway is missing, humoral transmission of the impulse may take its place. The latter mode of action is made possible by the existence of specialized areas within the central nervous system, i. e., the neurosecretory centers. The unique property of these centers lies in their dual capacity as nervous and glandular elements which allows the "translation" of afferent nervous impulses into efferent endocrine messages [E. SCHARRER (1952)]. Such neuro-endocrine chain reactions are well known in vertebrates. They also exist in invertebrates as, for instance, in insects. An analysis of the physiological events governing postembryonic development and reproduction in insects may serve to illustrate this point.

I. Growth and Metamorphosis

It is by now a well established fact that during postembryonic development in insects the target organs are under the influence of at least two different glands of internal secretion, the prothoracic glands (or their equivalents) and the corpora allata (Fig. 1). The eventual result, i. e., cessation of growth and

---

* Part of the work reported in this article was done under a grant from the American Cancer Society.

completion of adult development, is accomplished by a gradual shift in the relative importance of the two interacting hormone systems up to the point where only one of them, that resulting in the release of the prothoracic gland hormone, remains active. It is obvious that the delicate changes in hormone balance throughout this period necessitate an integrative mechanism to control the glands which produce these hormones. In this type of control mechanism it would seem advantageous for the two glands to share the same superior center. This center, in addition to "processing" the impulses intended for *each* gland, could also serve to correlate the activities of *both*. Although it has been known for some time that the corpora allata, as well as the prothoracic glands, are actually governed by the same neurosecretory center in the brain, the significance of this arrangement has never been analyzed.

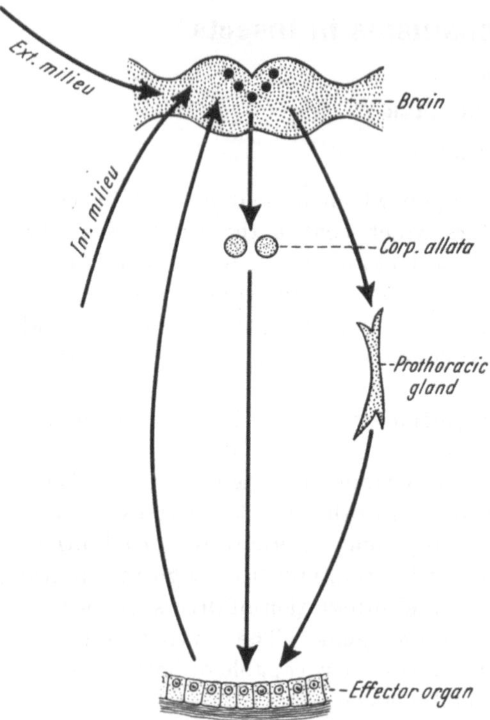

Fig. 1. Diagram illustrating the control of postembryonic development in insects. Two interacting hormone sources involved (prothoracic glands and corpora allata) are governed by the same integrative center in the brain which receives stimuli from internal and external milieu. Black circles in brain indicate neurosecretory cells. For further details see text

Let us now examine the manner in which this control takes place in each case. As has been shown by Williams (1952) and others, the function of the prothoracic glands depends on a hormone furnished by neurosecretory cells in the protocerebrum (pars intercerebralis and adjacent areas). Thus, at least in many groups of insects, a nervous connection need not and actually does not exist between this part of the brain and the prothoracic glands. The only known case in which the situation is somewhat different occurs in certain Diptera (see Possompès, this symposium, p. 96) and may be explained by the high degree of specialization reached in this group of insects. Generally speaking, whatever factors initiate or modify the action of the prothoracic gland (seasonal influences, nutritional status, etc.) presumably do so by acting on the neurosecretory center in the brain. These impulses are then integrated and transmitted to the prothoracic glands by means of a hormonal link. The manner in which the brain, in particular its neurosecretory components, controls the activity of the corpus allatum is less thoroughly understood. As will be discussed later (p. 82), there is evidence for both a restraining [B. Scharrer (1946a, 1952)] and a stimulating type of control.

Without going further into detail, it may be stated at this point that insect development is governed by a system of endocrine glands in whose over-all control a neurosecretory center within the brain plays a major role.

II. Reproduction

The central nervous system with its neurosecretory cells takes an equally important part in the control of reproductive processes in the female insect (Fig. 2). This situation will be discussed here largely on the basis of studies in the ovo-viviparous roach, *Leucophaea maderae*, a species which lends itself particularly well to such an analysis. Its reproductive cycle is characterized by a period of ovarian quiescence during the development of the embryos *in utero*. As in the majority of other insect species studied, the corpus allatum furnishes a "gonadotropic" hormone. In relation to various phases of the ovarian cycle, the corpus allatum shows cyclic changes in activity which also express themselves morphologically [ENGELMANN (1957)]. After the beginning of each cycle, i. e., during a period when the ovary as well as the accessory sex glands depend on the gonadotropic hormone [B. SCHARRER (1946b)], the corpus allatum enlarges and acquires a different histological appearance: The absolute and relative amount of cytoplasm rises and the concentration of the nuclei decreases. These changes are characteristic of the "active" gland. Shortly before ovulation the reverse process sets in, and as long as the ootheca stays in the uterus, when the ovary presumably receives no hormonal stimulation, the corpus allatum remains "inactive", a state characterized by its smaller size and the greater density of nuclear distribution.

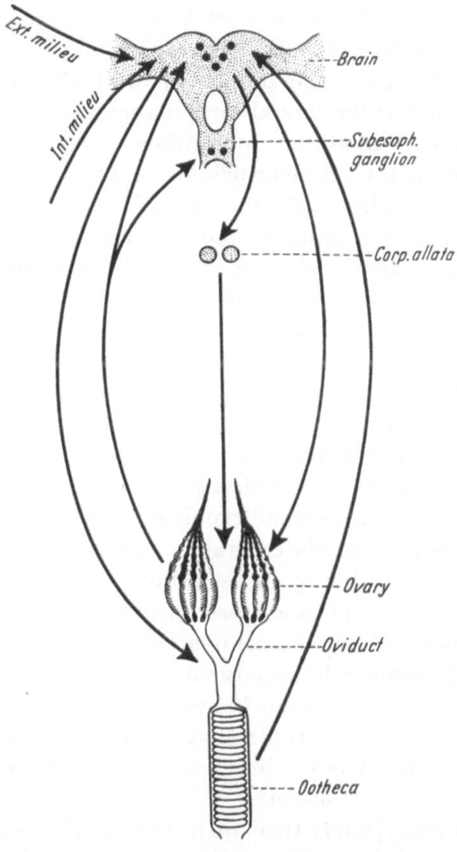

This rhythmicity is disturbed when the connection between corpora allata and brain is severed [B. SCHARRER (1952)]. The structure characteristic of the denervated corpus allatum resembles that of the "active" gland in the pre-ovulation phase, and the corpus allatum

Fig. 2. Diagram illustrating various factors controlling reproductive processes in adult female insects. The activity of the corpora allata (source of a gonadotropin) is governed by afferent stimuli from ovary and ootheca which are routed through the central nervous system. These and other modifying influences from internal and external milieu are integrated in the brain by means of neurosecretory cells (indicated by black circles). For further details see text

seems unable to return to the "inactive" state at the appropriate time. Even though the details of this situation still need to be worked out, one can conclude that, in the adult as well as in the developing insect, the corpus allatum is restrained in its activity by a superimposed center residing in the central nervous system. Furthermore, this restraining influence seems to take place at certain specific times during the reproductive cycle coinciding with the periods when the ovary receives no appreciable hormonal stimulation and therefore remains quiescent.

The question arises whether there are in addition any indications for the existence of a stimulation of the corpora allata by the brain. From experiments in adult flies *(Calliphora)*, E. Thomsen (1952) suggested the existence of an "allatotropic" hormone. More recently Nayar (this symposium, p. 102) postulated a similar situation in the bug *Iphita*, where he observed neurosecretory material entering the corpus allatum during a phase of the reproductive cycle in which the gland becomes active. The morphological conditions as known at present theoretically are consistent with the existence of more than one type of controlling pathway [Engelmann and Lüscher (1956)]. The corpora allata receive fibers from the brain (nervi corporis allati), a certain proportion of which originate in the neurosecretory cells of the pars intercerebralis and carry neurosecretory material. Thus stimuli from the brain to the corpus allatum can be either nervous or endocrine (neuro-hormonal). In the latter case, the active principle could reach the gland not only through the general circulation, but also more directly via the neurosecretory fibers. Which of these pathways are actually used and in which way, cannot be decided with certainty, but the existing evidence favors the supposition that the restraining influence on the corpus allatum takes place by nervous activity, whereas the stimulatory effect is brought about by a substance present in the neurosecretory material.

In this connection it is of interest to call attention to the observation in *Calliphora* [E. Thomsen (1952)] that the neurosecretory cells of the pars intercerebralis also exert direct endocrine control on the ovary, in this case bypassing the corpus allatum. It is perhaps no coincidence that this modification occurs in the same highly specialized insect that proved to be different with respect to the endocrine events governing postembryonic development (see Possompès, this symposium, p. 96). To summarize, the central nervous system participates in the endocrine control of the ovary either by its influence on the corpus allatum, or by its direct hormonal effect on the ovary (demonstrated in *Calliphora* only). In our analysis of the series of reactions which control ovarian function, we now have to examine those steps which determine the impulses dispatched by the brain. This inquiry depends to some extent on whether or not the central nervous system represents an obligatory way-station for all factors controlling the activity of the reproductive organs, or whether some of them act more directly, i. e., on the corpus allatum or even on the gonad itself.

It is reasonable to assume that external stimuli such as light [De Wilde (1955)] exert their influence via the brain and the corpus allatum. There is now increasing evidence that internal conditions also, such as changes in metabolism, do not act directly on the ovary. Thus Johansson (1954, 1955) has demonstrated, in *Leucophaea* as well as *Oncopeltus*, that the inability of starving females to produce mature eggs is due to incompetence of the corpus allatum and not, as formerly thought, of the ovary. The fact that egg development occurs under conditions of total starvation in animals whose corpus allatum is severed from the brain (Johansson, personal communication), suggests that the afferent impulse in the intact female reaches the corpus allatum via the brain. A comparable situation seems to exist concerning the effect on the ovary of metabolic changes caused by parasitism in the bee *Andrena* [Brandenburg (1956)].

Next we have to inquire into the manner by which corpus allatum activity is modified by messages from organs specifically concerned with reproduction. There is no information regarding a possible feed-back mechanism from one of the known target organs, the accessory sex glands. There seems, however, little doubt that the corpus allatum is kept "informed" about the physiological state of the ovary. This can be concluded from the effect of ovariectomy which, in a variety of species including *Leucophaea* [VON HARNACK and SCHARRER (1956)], may lead to abnormal enlargement of the corpora allata. By analogy with comparable observations in vertebrates, this can be interpreted as a sign of excessive compensatory efforts on the part of the corpora allata which, over a prolonged period of time, receive no confirmation from their target organ that it has been properly stimulated.

What is the nature of the messages dispatched by the ovary during certain phases of its cycle, and how do they reach their destination, the corpus allatum ? From a variety of indications speaking in favor of the existence of ovarian hormones among insects (for the most recent see NAYAR, this symposium, p. 102), and for lack of evidence to the contrary, one may assume that these stimuli are endocrine rather than nervous. These messages could reach the corpus allatum directly or, as has been indicated in the diagram (Fig. 2), by way of the brain. The latter pathway, although not proved, is strongly suggested by several facts: (1) The similarity between the histological changes in the corpus allatum after nerve severance and after gonadectomy becomes understandable, if one interprets the enlargement of the denervated corpus allatum as a result of the interruption of a normally existing pathway "ovary → brain → corpus allatum". Obviously the effect on the corpus allatum should be the same whether, in the absence of the ovary, a message is not dispatched or whether, with the connection between brain and corpus allatum interrupted, it cannot get through. (2) In a comparable situation, i. e., in the control of the oviduct of *Iphita* by the gonad (NAYAR, this symposium, p. 102), hormonal stimuli originating in the ovary are directed toward and perceived by the pars intercerebralis where they elicit a humoral response (Fig. 2). In this connection it is also of interest that a similar relationship between ovary and central nervous system could be demonstrated in *Leucophaea*. In this case a specific type of neurosecretory cells (B cells of subesophageal ganglion) show distinct cytological changes after castration [B. SCHARRER (1955, 1956)] probably in response to the persistent absence of a normally existing hormonal stimulation of this neurosecretory center by the ovary (Fig. 2). (3) If the stimuli from the ovary destined for the corpus allatum are routed through the brain, integration becomes possible with other messages which are known to pass through the central nervous system. Aside from external stimuli already mentioned, such as light, one specific case must be cited. There exists in *Leucophaea* a chain reaction "ootheca → brain → corpus allatum → ovary" (Fig. 2) by means of which the corpus allatum is prevented from stimulating the ovary as long as the developing embryos occupy the uterus [ENGELMANN (1957)]. This control mechanism is abolished after severance of the connections between brain and corpora allata, a result which demonstrates the existence of the "brain → corpus allatum" link. The endocrine stimulus from the ootheca seems to have precedence over the events dictated by the status of the ovary. Generally, the absence of large eggs permits the activation of the corpora allata which in turn initiates a cycle of ovarian growth. This is prevented by the ootheca during whose presence in the uterus ovulation could not take place. One can readily visualize that the activity of the ovary is the result of the integration in one strategic center of various influences either favoring or preventing the onset of a reproductive cycle. A great deal speaks in favor of localizing this center in the area of the neurosecretory cells of the brain.

In summary, the endocrine phenomena in insects selected for analysis in this paper should be viewed not so much as isolated events but rather as links in a system of chain reactions, part of which form closed circles. In this sequence of chain reactions the central nervous system constitutes a link of prime importance. It acts as an over-all controlling center in which nervous and endocrine stimuli from the external and internal milieu are assembled, integrated, and dispatched. The outgoing impulses are transmitted either to effector organs directly, or to glands of internal secretion which serve as way-stations. What deserves special emphasis here is the fact that the central nervous system is capable of dispatching not only nervous but also endocrine messages. This great versatility stems from the existence, within the central nervous system, of specialized centers of neurosecretory cells with their unique dual properties, and herein seems to lie the significance of the phenomenon of neurosecretion. Functional systems comparable to those discussed here in insects may be expected to exist in other groups of animals, i. e., in crustaceans and certain other invertebrates. The basic similarity to neuroendocrine mechanisms in vertebrates is evident from a recent analysis of the subject [Rothballer (1957)].

References

Brandenburg, J.: Das endokrine System des Kopfes von Andrena vaga PZ. (Ins. Hymenopt.) und Wirkung der Stylopisation (Stylops, Ins. Strepsipt.). Z. Morph. Ökol. Tiere **45**, 343—364 (1956).

Engelmann, F.: Die Steuerung der Ovarfunktion bei der ovoviviparen Schabe Leucophaea maderae (Fabr.). J. Insect Physiol. **1**, 257—278 (1957).

— and M. Lüscher: Die hemmende Wirkung des Gehirns auf die Corpora allata bei Leucophaea maderae (Orthoptera). Verh. dtsch. zool. Ges. (Hamburg) **1956**, 215—220.

Harnack, M. v., and B. Scharrer: A study of the corpora allata of gonadectomized Leucophaea maderae (Blattaria). Anat. Rec. **125**, 558 (1956).

Johansson, A. S.: Corpus allatum and egg production in starved milkweed bugs. Nature (Lond.) **174**, 89 (1954).

— The relationship between corpora allata and reproductive organs in starved female Leucophaea maderae (Blattaria). Biol. Bull. **108**, 40—44 (1955).

Rothballer, A. B.: Neuroendocrinology. Excerpta med. Sec. III, Endocrinology 11, 3-12 (1957).

Scharrer, B.: Section of the nervi corporis cardiaci in Leucophaea maderae (Orthoptera). Anat. Rec. **96**, 577 (1946a).

— The relationship between corpora allata and reproductive organs in adult Leucophaea maderae (Orthoptera). Endocrinology **38**, 46—55 (1946b).

— Neurosecretion XI. The effects of nerve section on the intercerebralis-cardiacum-allatum system of the insect Leucophaea maderae. Biol. Bull. **102**, 261—272 (1952).

— "Castration cells" in the central nervous system of an insect (Leucophaea maderae, Blattaria). Trans. N. Y. Acad. Sci., Ser. II, **17**, 520—525 (1955).

— Corrélations endocrines dans la reproduction des insectes. Ann. des Sci. Nat., Zool., 11e sér., **18**, 231—234 (1956).

Scharrer, E.: The general significance of the neurosecretory cell. Scientia (Milano), Ser. 6, **87**, 176—182 (1952).

Thomsen, E.: Functional significance of the neurosecretory brain cells and the corpus cardiacum in the female blow-fly, Calliphora erythrocephala Meig. J. exper, Biol. **29**, 137—172 (1952).

Wilde, J. de: The significance of the photoperiod for the occurrence of diapause in the adult Leptinotarsa decemlineata Say. Proc. 1st Internat. Photobiol. Congr. (1955).

Williams, C. M.: Physiology of insect diapause. IV. The brain and prothoracic glands as an endocrine system in the Cecropia silkworm. Biol. Bull. **103**, 120—138 (1952).

Laboratoire de Zoologie de la Sorbonne, Paris, France

Quelques aspects des phénomènes de neuro-sécrétion chez les Phasmides

Par

Marie Dupont-Raabe

Avec 6 Figures

L'étude des phénomènes de neuro-sécrétion chez les Phasmides, poursuivie récemment en collaboration avec mon élève, Mademoiselle Maurice, a permis observations diverses qui seront brièvement rapportées ici.

1. Phénomènes sécrétoires au niveau du tritocérébron

Des recherches expérimentales antérieures ont mis en évidence l'existence de phénomènes sécrétoires au niveau du tritocérébron des Phasmides, liés à la régulation de l'adaptation chromatique [Dupont-Raabe (1953, 1954)]. Rappelons brièvement que la commande du changement de coloration nycthéméral de ces Insectes est due à la libération dans le sang d'une substance d'origine cérébrale dont la localisation dans le cerveau a pu être précisée d'une part par des expériences d'ablation élective des régions neuro-sécrétrices protocérébrales, d'autre part par l'injection d'extraits effectués à partir de différentes portions du cerveau. L'ablation des régions neuro-sécrétrices protocérébrales, même lorsqu'elle s'accompagne d'une ablation des *corpora cardiaca*, laisse subsister une variation périodique normale ce qui indique que ces régions ne sont pas impliquées dans l'élaboration de la substance chromactive cérébrale. Des extraits de deux ou parfois trois portions séparées du cerveau ont été effectués selon des modalités différentes; ni la *pars intercerebralis*, ni la moitié postérieure protocérébrale du cerveau, ni la région médiane où se situe le trajet des *nervi corporis cardiaci* I ne sont actives; la substance chromactive est uniquement présente dans la région deuto- et tritocérébrale [Dupont-Raabe (1954, 1956*d, e*)].

Ces constatations expérimentales conduisaient à rechercher une traduction histologique de processus sécrétoires au niveau du deuto ou du tritocérébron. L'existence de phénomènes sécrétoires au niveau du tritocérébron n'apparaît qu'après l'utilisation de certaines techniques appropriées. Ainsi une fixation cytologique est indispensable; une coloration à la fuchsine d'Altmann sur du matériel postchromé ou une coloration à l'hématoxyline ferrique après fixation au Champy révèlent d'une part la présence de nombreuses flaques réparties dans la région fibreuse antéro-médiane du tritocérébron, d'autre part la présence de granulations dans une ou deux grandes cellules ventrolatérales [Dupont-Raabe (1954, 1956a)]. Les microphotographies 1 et 3 montrent l'aspect sous lequel se présentent ces cellules après une fixation et une coloration banale; les microphotographies 2 et 4 montrent ces mêmes cellules après une fixation cytologique et une coloration à l'azan. Cette coloration semble de beaucoup la technique la plus élective parmi celles utilisées jusqu'à présent. Elle permet de reconnaître aisément même à un faible grossissement la localisation d'une cellule sécrétrice tritocérébrale. A un grossissement plus fort, on distingue nettement la présence de nombreux grains de sécrétion

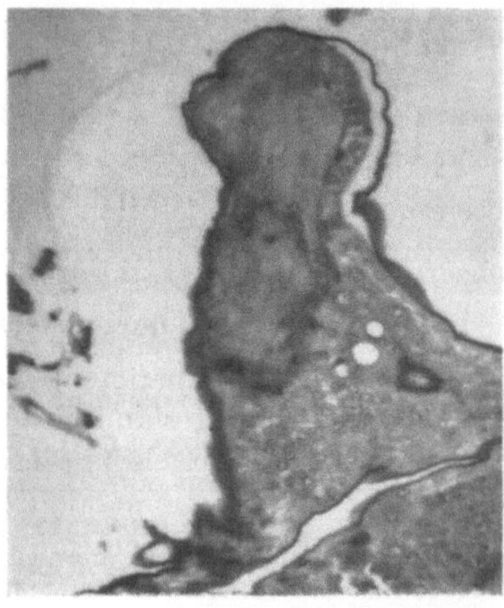

Fig. 1. Vue d'ensemble du cerveau montrant la position de la cellule sécrétrice tritocérébrale. Bouin, trichrome de Masson. La présence de produits de sécrétion n'est pas visible

Fig. 2. Aspect de la cellule sécrétrice tritocérébrale après fixation cytologique et coloration à l'azan

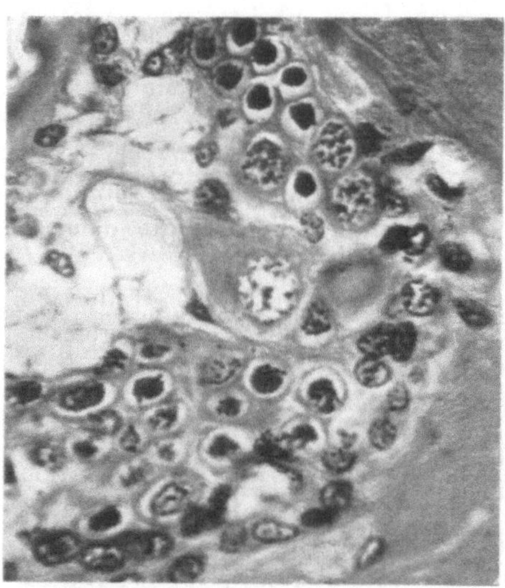

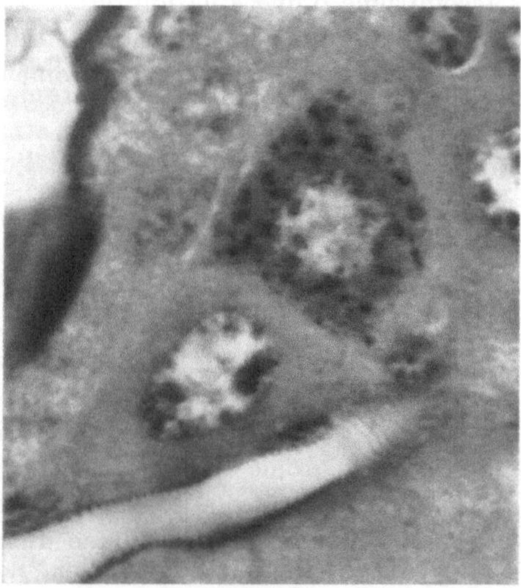

Fig. 3. Détail de la figure 1

Fig. 4. Détail de la figure 2. On peut observer la présence de nombreuses granulations intracytoplasmiques de forme irrégulière, répartis dans l'ensemble du cytoplasme. Sur certaines préparations, on peut même observer leur cheminement dans le large axone qui s'oriente vers la région antérieure du cerveau. Ni l'hématoxyline chromique, ni la fuchsine paraldéhyde ne colorent les granulations contenues dans ces cellules tritocérébrales. Elles mettent par contre en évidence de façon assez nette, les flaques présentes dans la région des fibres. Si celles-ci représentent, comme on peut le penser, le produit de sécrétion provenant des cellules sécrétrices tritocérébrales, il est plausible d'admettre que celui-ci subit, dans la partie distale des axones, certaines transformations qui augmentent sa colorabilité.

En ce qui concerne le problème de la destinée des produits de sécrétion tritocérébraux, des recherches expérimentales sur lesquelles il n'est pas possible de s'étendre ici, semblent indiquer que leur libération s'effectue au niveau du ganglion sous-œsophagien où l'on observe également la présence de flaques dans les régions fibreuses antéro-latérales [DUPONT-RAABE (1956c)]. Par ailleurs, on sait que les *corpora cardiaca* contiennent une substance chromactive A proche de la substance tritocérébrale mais non identique à celle-ci [DUPONT-RAABE (1952b, 1956b)]. On peut penser que la substance A est un produit de transformation de la substance tritocérébrale; elle pourrait parvenir du tritocérébron aux *corpora cardiaca* par la voie d'une troisième paire de *nervi corporis cardiaci* qui relie chez les Phasmides le tritocérébron aux *corpora cardiaca*.

2. Variabilité de comportement des différents produits de sécrétion cérébraux vis-à-vis des fixateurs et des colorants utilisés

L'emploi sur un même matériel de techniques de fixation et de coloration diverses fait apparaître clairement que tout au moins en ce qui concerne les Phasmides, les produits de sécrétion cérébraux se comportent de manière différente vis-à-vis des fixateurs et des colorants. Ainsi les produits de sécrétion de la *pars intercerebralis* sont bien conservés par les fixateurs aqueux et même alcooliques, alors que les produits de sécrétion des cellules protocérébrales latérales et du tritocérébron ne sont conservés qu'après l'emploi de fixateurs cytologiques [DUPONT-RAABE (1956a)]. Du point de vue des affinités tinctoriales, il est curieux de constater que si les cellules de la *pars intercerebralis* sont colorées de façon spectaculaire par l'hématoxyline chromique comme par la fuchsine paraldéhyde, les cellules protocérébrales latérales ne se distinguent que difficilement, par une certaine phloxinophilie de leur cytoplasma, après l'emploi de la technique de Gomori, mais apparaissent au contraire de façon très nette après utilisation de la fuchsine paraldéhyde qui colore franchement des grains cellulaires d'assez grande taille. Les produits de sécrétion tritocérébraux ont des affinités encore différentes comme on a pu le voir précédemment; la présence de granulations intracellulaires ne peut être mise en évidence ni par l'hématoxyline chromique ni par la fuchsine paraldéhyde, mais s'observe de façon très nette après coloration à l'azan.

Les conclusions qui découlent de ces observations semblent être qu'il existe au moins trois produits de sécrétion cérébraux différents, élaborés respectivement dans la *pars intercerebralis*, les cellules protocérébrales latérales et le tritocérébron. Rappelons en outre que certains éléments de la *pars intercerebralis* qui ne peuvent être distingués des autres après emploi de la fuchsine paraldéhyde, se colorent fortement, dans la technique de Gomori, par la phloxine et non par l'hématoxyline;

ils se rapprochent par là des cellules protocérébrales latérales. La réaction de Hotchkiss-MacManus de mise en évidence des polysaccharides semble révéler également une parenté entre ces deux types cellulaires.

3. Répercussions observées après section des nervi corporis cardiaci

Des sections des *nervi corporis cardiaci* au niveau de la partie tout à fait antérieure des *corpora cardiaca* ont été faites pour étudier, chez les Phasmides, les modalités de décharge des produits de sécrétion contenus dans ces organes, après l'interruption de leur innervation. On peut constater que la décharge s'effectue de façon assez lente: ainsi 10 jours après l'opération les *corpora cardiaca* des

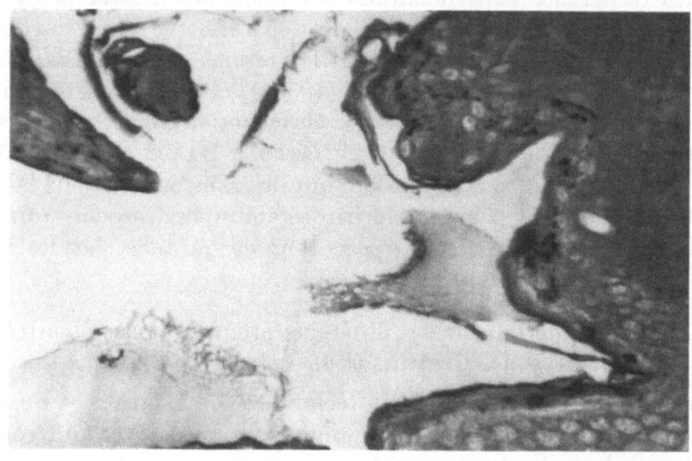

Fig. 5. Importante accumulation de flaques, fortement colorées par la fuchsine paraldéhyde, à la périphérie ventrale du cerveau chez un animal ayant subi deux mois auparavant une section des *nervi corporis cardiaci*

animaux opérés diffèrent peu de ceux d'animaux normaux, au bout d'un ou deux mois les différences sont au contraire assez frappantes et l'on trouve des images semblables à celles décrites par B. SCHARRER, chez la Blatte; les *corpora cardiaca* des animaux opérés sont presque totalement vidés de leurs produits de sécrétion; la partie proximale restée en liaison avec le cerveau semble au contraire hypertrophiée et contient de très nombreuses flaques: l'abondance des produits de sécrétion contenus dans la partie extra et intracérébrale des *nervi corporis cardiaci* et dans les cellules de la *pars intercerebralis* est considérablement augmentée, et ceci est particulièrement net chez une espèce comme *Carausius* où la neurosécrétion n'est jamais très intense.

Il faut signaler par ailleurs un fait assez surprenant qui a été observé de façon constante chez les animaux opérés; c'est une dispersion des produits de sécrétion dans l'ensemble du cerveau. Il semblerait que devant la difficulté d'écoulement des produits élaborés par les cellules neuro-sécrétrices, due à l'interruption de la liaison avec les *corpora cardiaca*, ceux-ci soient capables d'emprunter des voies nerveuses anormales; c'est ainsi que l'on rencontre en différentes régions du cerveau des traînées de flaques colorables par la fuchsine paraldéhyde et par l'hématoxyline chromique, accolées à divers faisceaux de fibres proto, deuto et tritocérébraux. Une accumulation importante des produits de sécrétion semble se faire par ailleurs à la périphérie du cerveau et notamment dans la partie ventrale de celui-ci; on observe une grande abondance de grains et de flaques dans les cellules même de la paroi du cerveau.

4. Réaction des polyphénols au niveau du ganglion frontal

La recherche des polyphénols au moyen de la réaction argentaffine, bien qu'elle ait donné des résultats négatifs en ce qui concerne le cerveau, a permis une constatation intéressante; en effet des résultats positifs nets ont pu être obtenus sur un élément du système sympathique, le ganglion frontal, dont les grandes cellules révèlent après l'emploi de cette technique la présence de nombreuses granulations colorées en noir par l'argent réduit. Ces granulations n'apparaissent pas après un traitement direct par le réactif de Schiff et ne correspondent donc pas à des fonctions aldéhydiques libres. Il se pourrait par conséquent que le système nerveux sympathique des Insectes contienne un polyphénol proche de l'adrénaline. Rappelons que la présence de produits de sécrétion dans le ganglion frontal des Insectes a été signalée chez différentes espèces mais leur signification physiologique demeurait obscure. Par ailleurs différents polyphénols: adrénaline, nor-adrénaline, dopamine et un quatrième orthodiphénol encore non identifié, le «catéchol-4»

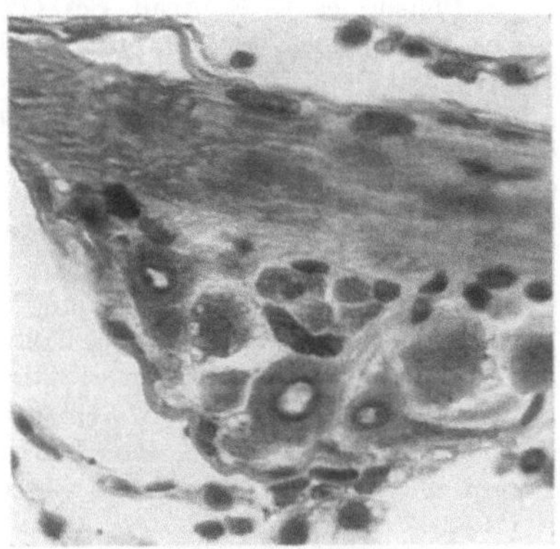

Fig. 6. Réaction argentaffine de mise en évidence des polyphénols. Les grandes cellules du ganglion frontal contiennent de nombreuses granulations argentaffines

ont pu être isolés par chromatographie du corps des Insectes [ÖSTLUND (1954)]. WIGGLESWORTH (1953) et CAMERON (1953) ont montré la présence dans les *corpora cardiaca* d'un orthodiphénol différent des corps actuellement connus et qui pourrait être le catéchol-4 d'ÖSTLUND. L'existence d'une réaction argentaffine nette au niveau du ganglion frontal fait penser que le système nerveux sympathique des Insectes est peut-être impliqué dans la production d'adrénaline, de nor-adrénaline ou de dopamine.

Bibliographie

CAMERON, M. L.: The secretion of an orthodiphenol in the *corpus cardiacum* of the Insect. Nature (Lond.) **172**, 349 (1953).

CARLISLE, D. B., M. DUPONT-RAABE et F. G. W. KNOWLES: Recherches préliminaires relatives à la séparation et à la comparaison des substances chromactives des Crustacés et des Insectes. C. R. Acad. Sci. (Paris) **240**, 665—667 (1955).

DE LERMA, B., M. DUPONT-RAABE et F. G. W. KNOWLES: Sur la question de la fluorescence des substances chromactives des Crustacés et des Insectes. C. R. Acad. Sci. (Paris) **241**, 995—998 (1955).

DUPONT-RAABE, M.: Etude expérimentale de l'adaptation chromatique chez le Phasme, *Carausius morosus*. C. R. Acad. Sci. (Paris) **232**, 886—888 (1951a).

— Etude morphologique et cytologique du cerveau de quelques Phasmides. Bull. Soc. Zool. France **76**, 5—6, 386—397 (1951b).

— Neuro-sécrétion chez les Phasmides. Bull. Soc. Zool. France **77**, 236 (1952a).

— Substances chromactives de Crustacés et d'Insectes. Activité réciproque, répartition. différences qualitatives. Arch. Zool. exp. gén. **89**, N. R. 3, 102—112 (1952b).

DUPONT-RAABE, M.: Le rôle endocrine du cerveau dans la régulation des phénomènes d'adaptation chromatique et de ponte chez les Phasmides. Pubbl. Staz. Zool. Napoli **24**, 63—66 (1953) (Symposium de Neurosécrétion).
— Répartition des activités chromatiques dans le ganglion sus-œsophagien des Phasmides: mise en évidence d'une région sécrétrice dans la partie deuto et tritocérébrale. C. R. Acad. Sci. (Paris) **238**, 950—951 (1954).
— Quelques données relatives aux phénomènes de neurosécrétion chez les Phasmides. Ann. Sci. Nat. Zool., 11° série, **18**, 2, 293—303 (1956a).
— Mise en évidence, chez les Phasmides, d'une troisième paire de *nervi corporis cardiaci*, voie possible de cheminement de la substance chromactive tritocérébrale vers les *corpora cardiaca*. C. R. Acad. Sci. (Paris) **243**, 1240—1243 (1956b).
— Rôle des différents éléments du système nerveux central dans la variation chromatique des Phasmides. C. R. Acad. Sci. (Paris) **243**, 1358—1360 (1956c).
— Les Mécanismes de l'adaptation chromatique chez les Insectes. Année biol. **32**, 7—8, 247—280 (1956d).
— Les Mécanismes de l'adaptation chromatique chez les Insectes. Arch. Zool. exp. gén. **94**, 61—293 (1956e).
KNOWLES, F. G. W., D. B. CARLISLE and M. DUPONT-RAABE: Studies on pigment activating substances in animals; I. The separation by paper electrophoresis of chromactivating substances in Arthropods. J. Mar. Biol. Ass. U. K. **34**, 611—635 (1955a).
— — — Inactivation enzymatique d'une substance chromactive des Insectes et des Crustacés. C. R. Acad. Sci. (Paris) **242**, 825 (1955b).
ÖSTLUND, E.: The distribution of catechol amines in lower animals and their effect on the heart. Acta physiol. scand. **31**, Suppl. 112, 1—67 (1954).
SCHARRER, B.: Neurosecretion XI. The effect of nerve section on the *intercerebralis-cardiacum-allatum* system of the insect, *Leucophaea maderae*. Biol. Bull. **102**, 261—272 (1952).
WIGGLESWORTH, V. B.: Neurosecretion and the *corpus cardiacum* of insects. Pubbl. Staz. Zool. Napoli **24**, 41—45 (1953).

Laboratoire de génétique évolutive, C.N.R.S., Gif sur Yvette, S et O, France

Le rôle des ptérines dans le mécanisme hormonal du complexe rétrocérébral chez les insectes

Par

Colette L'Hélias

Avec 1 Figure

Dans une étude précédente, la présence de substances photoréceptrices, les dérivés ptéridiniques, avaient pu être décélée dans la pars intercerebralis et le complexe rétrocérébral des Phasmes (*1*). Les substances extraites de ces organes par électrophorèse, réinjectées à ces animaux entraînent des modifications

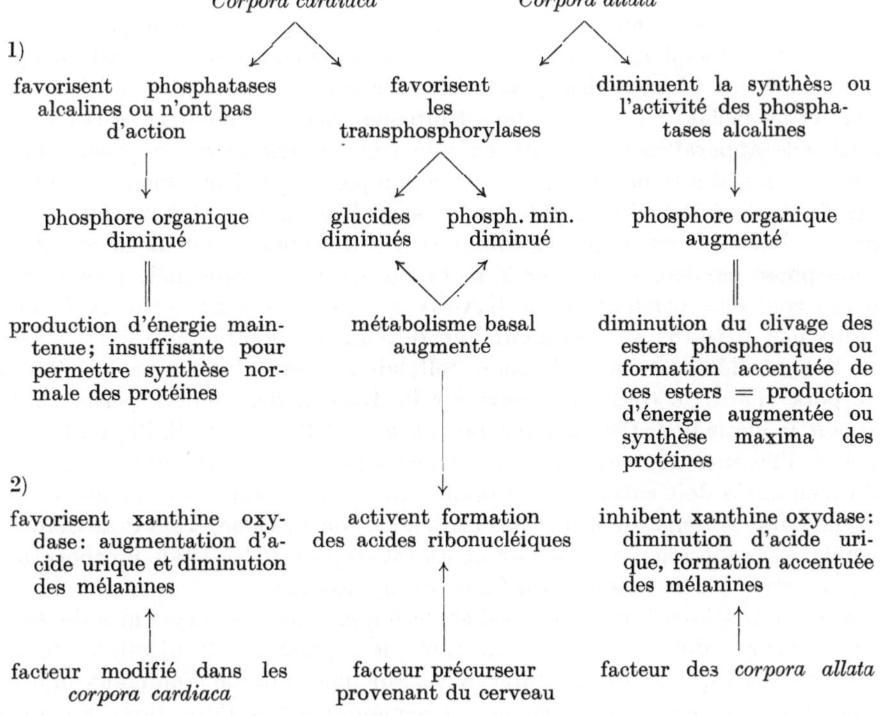

physiologiques importantes, de même que l'acide folique de synthèse. D'une part, elles provoquent des modifications pigmentaires chez les animaux opérés, mélanisation chez les cardiacotomisés, passage de la teinte jaune cuivrée à une couleur brun orangée de la cuticule chez les allatectomisés, d'autre part une accélération de la croissance dans le sens de la différenciation adulte. L'intermue si prolongé de l'allatectomisé est ramené à une durée normale. En même temps, l'étude biochimique de métabolisme m'avait permis de préciser l'action des substances hormonales du cerveau et du complexe rétrocérébral.

1) Un facteur photosensible est élaboré dans le cerveau et passe dans les corpora cardiaca par la voie nerveuse.

2) Dans les corpora cardiaca, ce facteur agit par lui-même ou plus vraisemblablement, se modifie partiellement pour constituer un premier facteur qui agit sur les sucres et les acides ribonucléiques. Cette action sur le métabolisme purique explique le rôle des corpora cardiaca dans la pigmentation: c'est, en effet, sur la xanthine oxydase que jouent ces organes et celle-ci est identique à la xanthoptérine oxydase qui transforme les ptérines. Les troubles provoqués chez celles-ci se répercutent sur les mélanines et les ommochromes qui s'accumulent et donnent une livrée gris argent à mouchetures noires au Phasme, lors de l'ablation des corpora cardiaca.

3) Une partie de ce précurseur du cerveau s'achemine jusqu'aux corpora allata et donne le deuxième facteur. Celui-ci agit sur les sucres et libère surtout l'énergie des liaisons phosphorées des esters glucidiques. L'énergie dégagée dans les réactions suffit pour provoquer la synthèse des protéines et explique donc le rôle des corpora allata dans la croissance du Phasme.

4) Sur la pigmentation, les corpora allata ont une réaction opposée à celle des c. cardiaca. Ces derniers provoquaient une augmentation de l'acide urique; eux, inversement, libèrent des quantités moindres de celui-ci; les ptérines sont oxydées et les mélanines, qui leur sont étroitement liées, augmentent. Aussi, l'ablation fait-elle apparaître une teinte cuivrée par disparition des pigments noirs.

Ces manifestations physiologiques et chimiques m'avaient amenées à penser que la formation des dérivés ptéridiniques ou l'association des ptérines et des hormones dans le cerveau et le complexe rétrocérébral excitent la glande de métamorphose par leur action sur le métabolisme et provoquent la prolifération cellulaire contrôlée pendant la vie larvaire par l'équilibre de ces deux facteurs ptéridiniques, naissant au détriment l'un de l'autre selon l'intensité de l'éclairement, l'un accélérateur de la division cellulaire, l'autre freinateur, sécrété par les corpora allata; le contrôle exercé sur la division des cellules permettant à celles-ci d'acquérir une structure spéciale et de se différencier. Si l'hypothése est exacte, en l'absence des corpora allata, dans les périodes d'inactivité, l'apport des ptérines en excès doit entraîner des proliférations désordonnées et même aboutir à des tumeurs. Aussi, ai-je utilisé des chrysalides de Pieridae, à l'état de diapause hivernale, où la sécrétion des corpora allata est stoppée et la glande prothoracique rendue inactive par la présence du facteur diapausant.

J'ai donc pratiqué les injections d'acide folique sur des chrysalides de *Pieris brassicae*; venant de se nymphoser au mois de septembre. 2 injections de $10\,\gamma$ furent répétées à quinze jours d'intervalle. Sur une centaine d'animaux injectés, une vingtaine meurent un mois ou six semaines après l'injection; les autres meurent tous trois mois plus tard, en quelques jours. Les animaux disséqués révèlent des désordres graves, présence de mélanoma noirs; localisés d'abord au point de l'injection (bas du thorax), puis se ramifiant dans l'abdomen et métastases péricardiales.

1) La tumeur primaire, développée au point de l'injection, se ramifie dans le thorax et les tissus voisins. L'épithélium et le corps gras sont envahis par les pigments mélaniques et dégénèrent. Ces ramifications donnent lieu à des proliférations locales le long du vaisseau dorsal, d'une part à partir des éléments

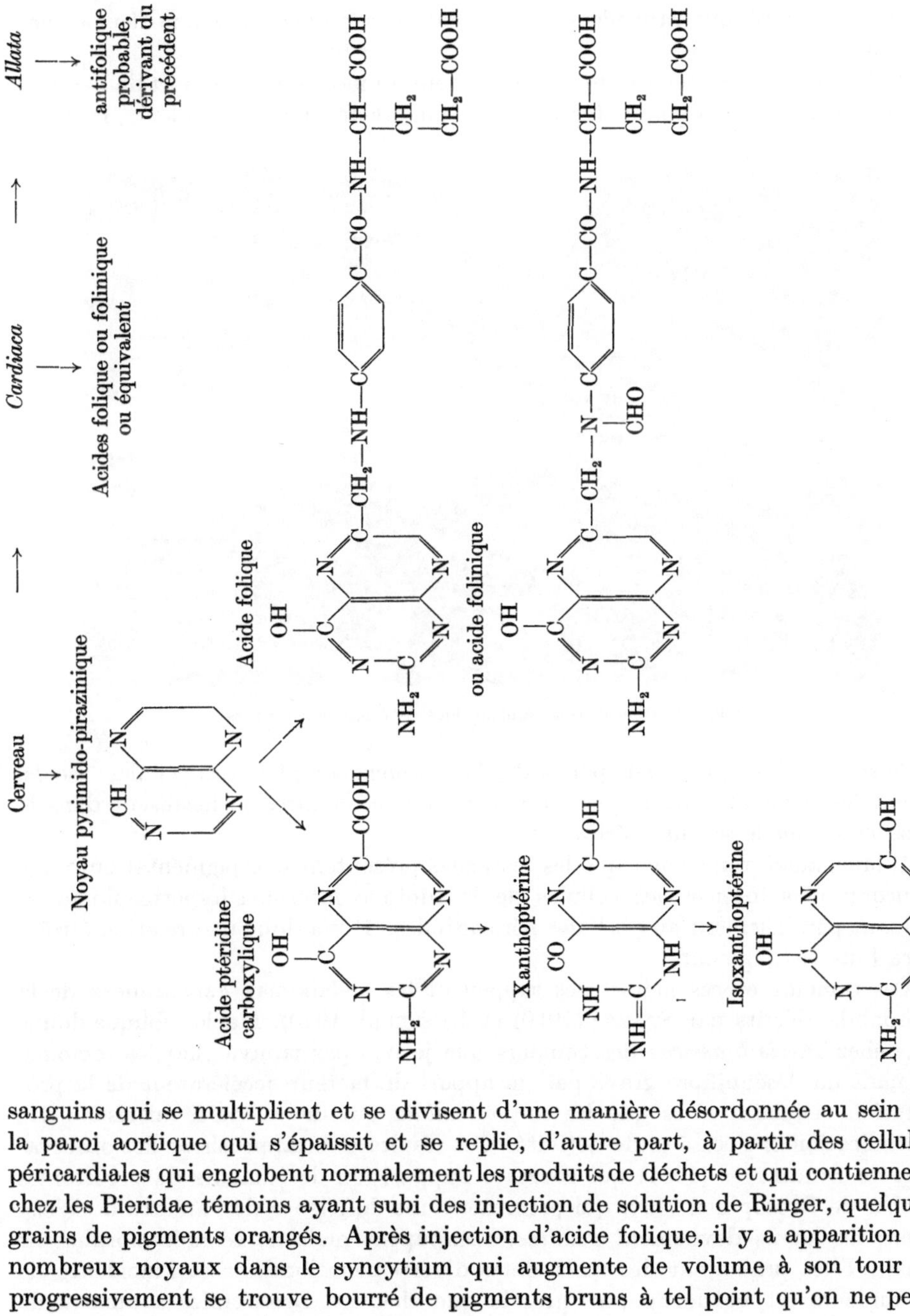

sanguins qui se multiplient et se divisent d'une manière désordonnée au sein de la paroi aortique qui s'épaissit et se replie, d'autre part, à partir des cellules péricardiales qui englobent normalement les produits de déchets et qui contiennent chez les Pieridae témoins ayant subi des injection de solution de Ringer, quelques grains de pigments orangés. Après injection d'acide folique, il y a apparition de nombreux noyaux dans le syncytium qui augmente de volume à son tour et progressivement se trouve bourré de pigments bruns à tel point qu'on ne peut plus apercevoir de cytoplasme libre, puis il y a formation de noyaux énormes, ronds ou plurilobés par fusion des petits noyaux ou par endomitose. Le volume de ces géants peut dépasser 10 à 15 fois la taille normale. Le syncytium acquiert les proportions correspondantes et se replie en lobes multiples et tourmentés si bien que l'ensemble des cellules péricardiales, le long du vaisseau dorsal, prend un aspect foliacé qui rappelle curieusement le sarcome en «chou-fleur» chez l'homme.

2) Les mélanomas secondaires se présentent au moment de la mort de l'animal sous forme de morulas pigmentées de brun, masses acellulaires d'ailleurs, la phase

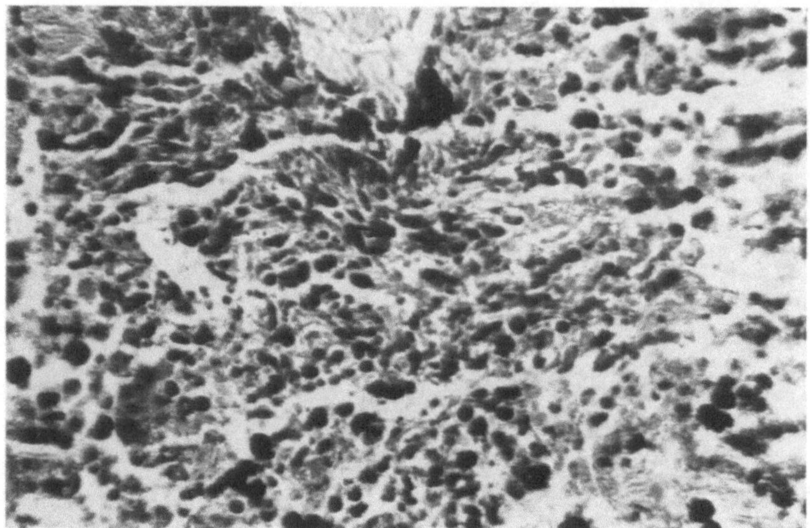

Fig. 1. Tumeur dans la paroi aortique. — Amas de leucocytes

finale se traduisant, en effet, par la dégénérescence complète des cellules. Seuls, restent les pigments mélaniques. Ces tumeurs secondaires se localisent dans le corps gras, sous le septum péricardial.

Il faut, aussi, remarquer que les testicules présentent une pigmentation rouge beaucoup plus intense, les cellules de la tunique interne s'hypertrophiant et évoluant parallélement aux cellules péricardiales. Il y a donc une relation étroite entre tous ces pigments.

Ces tumeurs et ces métastases rappellent les mélanomas «spontanés» de la Drosophile, décrits par Stark[6] (1919) et Russell[4] (1940). L'acide folique donne donc chez *Pieris brassicae* des tumeurs que je n'ai pas trouvé chez les témoins, amenant un déséquilibre grave par un apport de facteur accélérateur de la prolifération cellulaire alors que les *corpora allata* qui devraient régulariser cette multiplication ont cessé toute activité. Ces résultats se rapprochent des observations de Burdette[1] (1954) qui constate l'apparition de tumeurs dans certaines souches de Drosophiles *(tu)*, qui présentent une déficience de l'anneau de Weismann; les larves deviennent géantes, s'empupent mais ne se métamorphosent jamais. Elles présentent des melanomas diversement localisés et l'incidence de ces tumeurs est beaucoup plus grande que chez les Drosophiles à anneau de

Weismann normal. De même, PFLUGFELDER[3] (1938) par ablation des corpora allata chez *Dixippus morosus* et B. SCHARRER[5] (1948) par section des nerfs sympatiques chez *Leucophaea maderae* provoquaient la prolifération de certains tissus chez les animaux opérés.

Deux faits se dégagent de ces expériences:

1) L'acide folique suffit pour entrainer un processus pathologique chez des chrysalides en diapause, ce qui prouve que les ptérines jouent un rôle de première importance dans le déclanchement de la division cellulaire. It faut souligner que ce déclanchement des tumeurs par l'acide folique est bien lié à la diapause. En effet, des injections d'acide folique pratiquées chez *Galleria mellonella* qui ne présente pas de diapause, n'ont pas empêché les chrysalides de se développer normalement (injections faites au dernier stade larvaire, éclosion de l'imago trois semaines plus tard). Des injections d'acide folique pratiquées chez des chrysalides de *Pieris brassicae* à la fin de la diapause hivernale, au mois d'avril ne provoquent plus l'apparition de ces tumeurs, mais au contraire, un développement normal.

2) La présence de ptérines dans le complexe rétrocérébral, dans les régions neurosécrétrices du cerveau, les modifications qu'entraînent ces substances dans le métabolisme en contrôlant, en particulier, la synthèse des acides nucléiques, lorsqu'on les injecte à des Phasmes cardiaco- ou allatectomisés montrent qu'elles sont liées directement aux neurosécrétions du complexe rétrocérébral, donc au contrôle hormonal de la croissance, sans que je puisse préciser pour l'instant si ces relais photorécepteurs sont des intermédiaires chimiques permettant la biosynthèse des hormones ou s'ils sont eux-mêmes des co-hormones. Ces facteurs dérivant les uns des autres, exercent une activité d'antimétabolites et leur compétition maintient l'équilibre organique de l'animal qui permet à celui-ci de mener à bien sa croissance. Lorsque l'équilibre est rompu par la suppression de l'un des facteurs ou l'apparition d'un excès de facteur voisin, on passe du processus normal de division cellulaire à une prolifération anarchique des tissus. *De plus, les propriétés photoréceptrices de ces ptérines peuvent expliquer les variations normales du métabolisme* qui *suit le rythme des saisons*. L'allongement du jour, l'intensité plus forte de lumière font apparaître certains facteurs au détriment de ceux synthétisés dans l'obscurité modifiant ainsi le rapport de ces antimétabolites et l'intervention de facteurs extérieurs trop violents (chaleur, lumière, ultra-violets) peut entraîner par modifications de l'équilibre de ces ptérines les proliférations pathologiques de certains tissus. La présence de substances photosensibles dans le complexe *pars intercerebralis-cardiaca-allata* est peut-être la clé des stimulis qui déclanchent les réactions en chaîne cancérigènes et le parallélisme qui existe entre le complexe rétrocérébral et le système hypothalamo-hypophysaire des Vertébrés permettrait sans doute de généraliser cette hypothèse.

Bibliographie

1. BURDETTE, W. J.: Nat. Canc. Inst. **15**, 367 (1954).
2. L'HELIAS: C. R. Acad. Sci. (Paris) **240**, 1114—1116 (1955).
3. PFLUGFELDER, O.: Wiss. Zool. **152**, 159—184 (1938).
4. RUSSEL, E.: J. exp. Zool. **84**, 362 (1940).
5. SCHARRER, B., and M. S. LOCHHEAD: Cancer Res. **10**, no. 7 (1950).
6. STARK, M.: Proc. nat. Acad. Sci. (Wash.) **5**, 573 (1919).

Faculté des Sciences, Sorbonne, Paris V^e, France

Evolution des cellules neuro-sécrétrices protocérébrales et de la glande péritrachéenne de Calliphora erythrocephala Meig (Diptère) après section des connexions nerveuses entre le cerveau et l'anneau de Weismann

Par

B. Possompès

La section des nerfs d'origine cérébrale desservant l'anneau de Weismann, effectuée avant un moment critique donné du dernier stade larvaire libre de *Calliphora erythrocephala*, a pour effet la suppression de la métamorphose[1]. Une telle opération équivaut ainsi à une ablation de l'anneau de Weismann et entraîne le maintien à l'état de larve « permanente » [2].

L'action stimulatrice exercée par les cellules neuro-sécrétrices protocérébrales sur les grandes cellules de la glande péritrachéenne, composant de l'anneau de Weismann sécréteur de l'hormone de mue, requiert donc l'intégrité des nerfs unissant cerveau et anneau de Weismann [Possompès (1950, 1953a, b)].

L'exigence d'une telle continuité nerveuse est une modalité spéciale aux Diptères Cyclorrhaphes[3]. Elle conduit à penser que le facteur issu de la *pars intercerebralis* emprunte les voies nerveuses d'origine cérébrale desservant l'anneau de Weismann, c'est-à-dire les nerfs du *corpus cardiacum*[4], et parvient ainsi à la glande péritrachéenne anatomiquement solidaire du *corpus cardiacum*. La présente étude, associant expérimentation et cytologie, permet d'apporter quelques arguments en faveur d'une telle interprétation.

Sur des larves du dernier stade libre encore en période de digestion du contenu du jabot, les connexions cerveau-anneau de Weismann sont sectionnées et, en conséquence, l'état larve « permanente » se trouve réalisé. Une semaine environ après l'opération, c'est à dire nettement au-delà du moment où le sujet se serait

---

[1] Burtt (1939) avait constaté un effet analogue chez *C. vomitoria* après interruption de l'innervation de l'anneau de Weismann effectuée environ 4 jours avant la formation du puparium.

[2] La période critique au-delà de laquelle la rupture nerveuse devient inefficace précède notablement dans le temps la période critique d'action de l'anneau de Weismann lui-même (âge maximum auquel l'ablation de cette dernière formation empêche la métamorphose).

[3] Chez le Lépidoptère *Platysamia* [Williams (1947)] et chez l'Hémiptère *Rhodnius* [Wigglesworth (1951)], au contraire, le cerveau stimule la glande productrice de l'hormone de mue en l'absence de toute innervation de cette dernière.

[4] A la suite des travaux de B. et E. Scharrer (1944, etc....), de nombreuses recherches cytologiques ont mis en évidence, chez des Insectes variés, l'existence, le long des axones des nerfs des *C. cardiaca*, de produits figurés de neuro-sécrétion issus de la *pars intercerebralis* du protocerebrum [voir Gabe (1954)].

normalement empupé, ce dernier est sacrifié et traité suivant la technique de Gomori (hématoxyline chromique-phloxine).

a) Les cellules neuro-sécrétrices du protocerebrum manifestent des signes visibles d'une intense activité sécrétoire; leur cytoplasme est surchargé de produits de sécrétion basophiles intensément colorés par l'hématoxyline. Les images observées, comparées à des préparations relatives à des animaux témoins, semblent traduire une accumulation de substances vraisemblablement non évacuées en raison de la destruction des nerfs du *corpus cardiacum*.

b) La glande péritrachéenne de l'anneau de Weismann est réduite à un état évident de régression et de non fonctionnement: cytoplasme peu abondant, considérablement diminué à certains niveaux où les noyaux, normaux en apparence, se trouvent tassés les uns près des autres. Une comparaison avec la même formation observé chez des larves témoins permet de mesurer l'atrophie consécutive à l'opération.

Il paraît légitime de conclure à une corrélation entre les trois ordres de faits observés à la suite des opérations de rupture nerveuse effectuées dans ces expériences:

la rétention du produit protocérébral de neuro-sécrétion,

l'atrophie essentiellement cytoplasmique des cellules de la glande péritrachénne et la suppression de la métamorphose.

Nous connaissons parfaitement, du point de vue morphologique, la neuro-sécrétion à l'intérieur du système *pars intercerebralis — corpus cardiacum — corpus allatum* de nombreux Insectes, mais nous ignorons encore sa signification physiologique exacte. Les données morphologiques relatives à la production de substances neuro-sécrétées protocérébrales et les données expérimentales concernant le rôle du cerveau dans l'induction de la métamorphose de *Calliphora erythrocephala* permettent d'entrevoir les bases cytologiques des relations fonctionnelles entre la *pars intercerebralis* et la glande sécrétrice de l'hormone de mue des Diptères supérieurs.

Bibliographie

Burtt, E. T.: On the *corpora allata* of dipterous insects. II. Proceedings of the Royal Society of London, Series B. **126**, 210—223 (1939).

Gabe, M.: La neuro-sécrétion chez les Invertébrés. Année biol. **30**; 5—62 (1954).

Possompès, B.: Rôle du cerveau au cours de la métamorphose de *Calliphora erythrocephala* Meig. C. R. Acad. Sci. (Paris) **231**, 594—596 (1950).

— Recherches expérimentales sur le déterminisme de la métamorphose de *Calliphora erythrocephala* Meig. Arch. Zool. exp. gén. **89**, 203—364 (1953a).

— Les données expérimentales sur le déterminisme endocrine de la croissance des Insectes. Bull. Soc. Zool. France **78**, 240—275 (1953b).

Scharrer, B.: Neurosecretion XI. The effects of nerve section on the *intercerebralis-cardiacum-allatum* system of the Insect *Leucophaea maderae*. Biol. Bull. **102**, 261—272 (1952).

— et E. Scharrer: Neurosecretion VI. A comparison between the *intercerebralis-cardiacum-allatum* system of the Insects and the hypothalamo-hypophyseal system of the Vertebrates. Biol. Bull. **87**, 242—251 (1944).

Wigglesworth, V. B.: Sources of moulting hormone in *Rhodnius*. Nature (Lond.) **168**, 558 (1951).

Williams, C. M.: Physiology of Insect diapause. II. Interaction between the pupal brain and prothoracic glands in the metamorphosis of the giant silk worm, *Platysamia cecropia*. Biol. Bull. **93**, 89—98 (1947).

Zoological Laboratory, University of Oslo, Norway

Neurosecretion in the Milkweed Bug, Oncopeltus fasciatus (Dallas)

By

Arne S. Johansson

With 5 Figures

The milkweed bug, *Oncopeltus fasciatus* (DALLAS), has proved very favorable for histological and experimental studies on neurosecretion. The present paper gives a summary of what has been observed in this insect.

Neurosecretory cells are especially prominent in the pars intercerebralis region of the brain (Fig. 1). After the use of Gomori's aldehyde-fuchsin technique, as modified by HALMI and DAWSON, four types of rather large neurones can be identified in this region. The most conspicuous type is represented by two groups of 5 cells each. These cells, which probably correspond to the A cells described by NAYAR (1955) in the heteropteran *Iphita*, stain dark purple in aldehyde-fuchsin and blue-black in Gomori's chrome-hematoxylin-phloxin. The cell body is more or less filled with granules. Owing to their bluish-white colour these cells can be identified in the living animal.

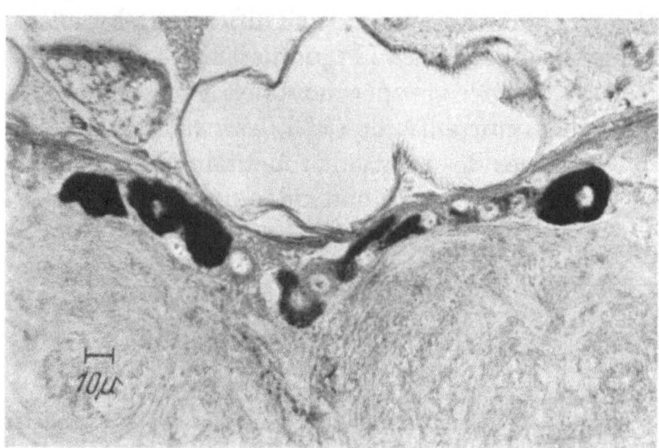

Fig. 1. Neurosecretory cells in the pars intercerebralis region of the brain. Helly. Aldehyde-fuchsin

Another type of neurone, found in the same area, is somewhat smaller and stains green in aldehyde-fuchsin and red in Gomori's chrome-hematoxylin-phloxin. These cells probably correspond to the B cells described by NAYAR in *Iphita* and KÖPF (1957) in *Drosophila*. Their number has not been determined with certainty.

A third type of neurone appears mixed in with the B cells. They have a flaky appearance, stain purplish in aldehyde-fuchsin and pale red in Gomori's chrome-hematoxylin-phloxin. They are of about the same size as the B cells and occur in the number of about 10.

The fourth type is situated in the median line and is slightly bigger than the A cells. They occur in the number of 4, have a pearshaped body, stain pale purplish in aldehyde-fuchsin, and do not show any special affinities to Gomori's chrome-hematoxylin-phloxin.

These four types of neurones have been identified in sexually mature adult males and females. The B cells are more difficult to stain, and in some preparations only the A cells show up.

Four single cells, somewhat smaller but otherwise much like the A cells of the brain, are present in the prothoracic ganglion. In the last composite ganglion, 14 similar cells are found. No such neurosecretory cells have been observed in the suboesophageal, the frontal or the hypocerebral ganglia.

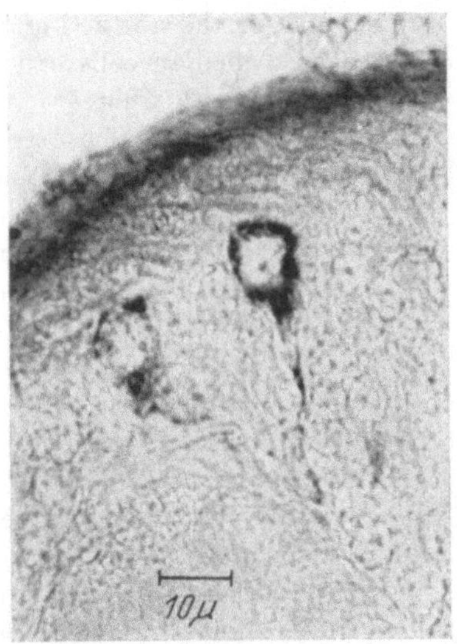

Fig. 2. Neurosecretory cells from the brain. Bouin.
Aldehyde-fuchsin

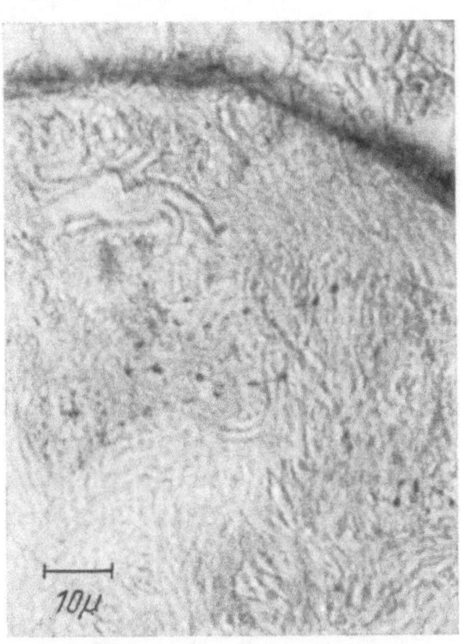

Fig. 3. Fibers with purple swellings in the prothoracic ganglion. Bouin. Aldehyde-fuchsin

In the most successful preparations, some of the neurones in various regions of all ganglia of the central nervous system stain more or less dark purplish, in contrast to the ordinary neurones (Fig. 2). The granulated content of these cells can be traced into the axon. Such cells, mostly small- and medium-sized association neurones, occur singly or in small groups and seem to have individual cycles of secretory activity. Similar observations have not been made among the globuli cells in the optic ganglia or the mushroom bodies, or among the large motor neurones in the ventral chain. In the same preparations, where these neurosecretory cells show up, moniliform fibers with purple swellings are found in the neuropile of all ganglia of the central nervous system (Fig. 3). It is assumed that these fibers belong to the purple neurones.

Distinct neurosecretory pathways are indicated by the presence of the granulated material in the axons from the 10 A cells in the pars intercerebralis. These axons cross over to the opposite side and leave the brain from the posterior region. They form the nervi corporis cardiaci I. The granulated material can be traced along the axons to the walls of the aorta where the material is found in lumps of various sizes (Fig. 4) as already described in *Iphita* [Nayar (1956)]. These accumulations are bluish in the living aorta when observed in darkfield illumination. In *Oncopeltus* no such material is observed in the corpora cardiaca-allata, and it seems as if the regions of the aorta adjacent to the corpora cardiaca-allata act as storage organ for this neurosecretory material.

Examination of nymphs showed that the 10 A cells are present already in the first instar, as is the neurosecretory material in the walls of the aorta (Fig. 5). The 4 median cells can be recognized whereas the other types of neurosecretory neurones in the pars intercerebralis have not been observed with our technique. The prothoracic and the last ganglion contain the same number, viz. 4 and 14, of neurosecretory cells in the first instar as in the adult.

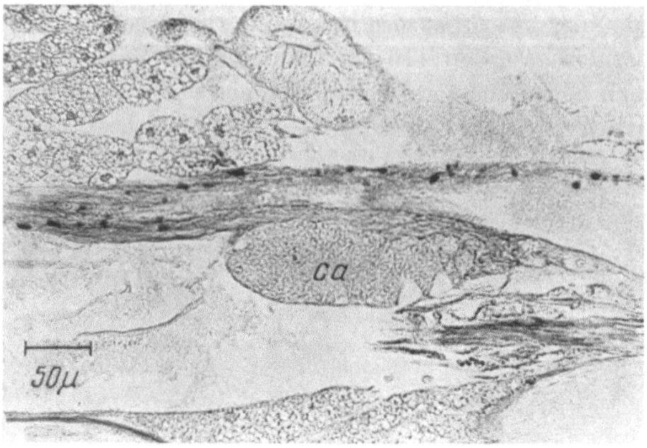

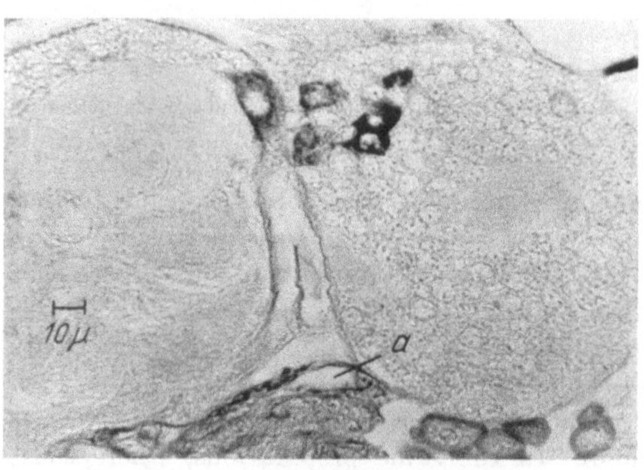

Fig. 4. Neurosecretory material in the walls of the aorta. *ca:* corpus allatum. Bouin. Aldehyde-fuchsin

Neurosecretory cells in the pars intercerebralis region have been found to be the source of the initial hormonal stimulus to molting and metamorphosis in various insects. In order to test their role in *Oncopeltus*, the neurosecretory cells of the protocerebrum were extirpated in 67 fifth stage nymphs shortly after the preceding molt. Twenty-three of the operated animals survived and molted again. Sectioned material, stained with aldehyde fuchsin, showed that specimens, which had their A cells as well as the other types of neurosecretory cells successfully extirpated as early as 4 hours after the preceding molt, were capable of molting.

Fig. 5. Neurosecretory cells in the brain of the first stage nymph. *a:* aorta with neurosecretory material in the walls. Bouin. Aldehyde-fuchsin

In another series of experiments, the possible role of the pars intercerebralis in the endocrine control of ovarian function was tested, since such a role had been demonstrated in at least one case, i. e., *Calliphora*, by Thomsen (1952). The A cells were extirpated in 149 females and 59 males of *Oncopeltus* varying in "adult age" from less than one hour to two days. Forty-eight females and 18 males survived the operation for a sufficient period of time. The reproductive organs of the males appeared normal. Forty-three of the females produced mature eggs, as did females which had all A cells extirpated in the fifth stage.

The negative results in both series of experiments do not necessarily prove that neurosecretory substances play no role in postembryonic development and reproduction of *Oncopeltus*. As E. and B. SCHARRER (1954, p. 1054) have pointed out, extirpation of the neurosecretory cells alone need not lead to drastic deficiencies in animals in which the storage of neurosecretory material in organs distant from the cells plays an important role.

As has been stated above, in *Oncopeltus* neurosecretory material is stored in the wall of the aorta. Its depletion from this site has been observed during metamorphosis (last molt) in normal nymphs as well as animals deprived of their neurosecretory cells. In other words, it seems that neurosecretory material can be mobilized at the site of storage even in the absence of the neurosecretory cells in which it originated. Theoretically at least, this observation is consistent with the view that neurosecretory material participates in the endocrine control of molting and metamorphosis in *Oncopeltus*.

By contrast, such a possibility must be ruled out for the control of reproductive processes. In the adult stages investigated, no relationship between the presence or absence of neurosecretory material in the aortic wall and ovarian function could be demonstrated. More significantly, females whose A cells had been removed already in the 5th nymphal stage and in which no storage of neurosecretory material occurred after they had reached the adult stage, were still capable of producing mature eggs. One might conclude that in *Oncopeltus* the endocrine control of ovarian function is carried out by other types of neurosecretory cells or by the corpus allatum alone. However, in females deprived of their A cells the corpus allatum was usually found to be of subnormal size, an observation which agrees with that of THOMSEN (1952) in *Calliphora*. Further experiments will have to elucidate the endocrine mechanisms controlling reproduction in *Oncopeltus*, as well as determine the functional role of neurosecretory substances in this insect.

Literature

KÖPF, H.: Zur Topographie und Morphologie neurosekretorischer Zentren bei Drosophila. Naturwissenschaften **44**, 121—122 (1957).

NAYAR, K. K.: Studies on the neurosecretory system of Iphita limbata Stal. I. Distribution and structure of the neurosecretory cells of the nerve ring. Biol. Bull. **108**, 296—307 (1955).

— Studies on the neurosecretory system of Iphita limbata Stal. III. The endocrine glands and the neurosecretory pathways in the adult. Z. Zellforsch. **44**, 697—705 (1956).

SCHARRER, E., and B. SCHARRER: Neurosekretion. Handbuch der mikroskopischen Anatomie des Menschen Bd. 6 (5), S. 953—1066 (1954).

THOMSEN, E.: Functional significance of the neurosecretory brain cells and the corpus cardiacum in the female blow-fly, Calliphora erythrocephala Meig. J. exp. Biol. **29**, 137—172 (1952).

Department of Zoology, University College, Trivandrum, India*

Probable Endocrine Mechanism Controlling Oviposition in the Insect Iphita Limbata Stal

By

K. K. NAYAR

With 1 Figure

Iphita limbata Stal (Pyrrhocoridae, Hemiptera) is a plant bug commonly occurring in South India. Histophysiological and experimental studies in adult females have shown that the ovary as well as the neurosecretory cells of the pars intercerebralis of the brain play a role in the control of oviposition.

I. Histological Studies

GOMORI's chrome alum hematoxylin phloxin method was used to demonstrate the presence of neurosecretory material during various phases of the reproductive cycle. In the newly emerged female very little stainable material is present in the cytoplasm of the neurosecretory cells of the pars intercerebralis. As feeding starts and the animal becomes rather active, many neurosecretory cells show inclusions staining dark blue. The same picture is maintained throughout the period of mating. When the behavior typical of the pre-oviposition period is observed (attempts to disengage the male by tapping it with the hindlegs, raising of rostrum, salivation, search with lowered antennae for sites suitable for egg laying, avoidance of male), a gradual decrease of stainable material occurs in the neurosecretory cells of the brain. At the time of oviposition, the blue staining material has disappeared from the cells which now contain phloxinophilic inclusions. Blue material starts to reappear during the period of rest which follows oviposition. These observations concur with those made earlier by DUPONT-RAABE (1951, 1952) in phasmids.

The growth and maturation of the ova in each reproductive cycle are accompanied not only by the changes in the pars intercerebralis just described, but also by cyclic changes in the volume of the corpus allatum, comparable to those known in other insect species. In the early phases of this cycle, the nervi corporis cardiaci and allati are devoid of neurosecretory material, but at the start of mating blue staining material can be traced all along the axons into the corpus allatum which then begins to enlarge. This observation may indicate an activation of this gland by neurosecretory material taking place at specific times of the reproductive cycle, and not at others. It is of particular interest that during the pre-oviposition period, when the corpus allatum contains no neurosecretory inclusions, these seem to leave the nervous pathway in the region of the corpora

---

* Present address: Government Victoria College, Palghat, South India

cardiaca to enter into the aorta. At the time of oviposition the nervi corporis cardiaci and allati lack neurosecretory material; it begins to reappear in the axons when mating occurs again.

II. Experimental Studies

Three types of experiments were performed.

(1) Blood transfusions were made by collecting hemolymph from amputated antennae into the needle of a fine syringe and injecting it in amounts of 0.05 to 0.1 ml. Blood from a donor showing beginning signs of pre-oviposition behavior induced egg deposition within 1—3 hours in females which were not yet ready to do so when left untreated. The same result was obtained with blood from a laying female or one which had just finished laying. By contrast, blood from younger donors, or from donors mating for the second time, did not bring about this effect.

These experiments indicate that oviposition in *Iphita* is induced by a blood borne factor. A comparable result was reported by MOKIA [vide SCHARRER (1955)] who induced oviposition by blood transfusion in *Bombyx*. In order to determine the source of this humoral factor in *Iphita*, further experiments were carried out.

(2) Aqueous extracts from ovaries in amounts of 0.1 to 0.2 ml were injected into the prothorax of females which were not ready to lay their eggs. Extracts prepared from ovaries containing mature eggs initiated pre-oviposition behavior and led to the premature laying of eggs. In some cases where the eggs of the recipients were still relatively small, these did not succeed in laying them. Instead, further egg development was stopped, and signs of degeneration were observed in these ovaries. The degenerative changes may have something to do with the depletion of neurosecretory material observed in these experimental animals at a stage where the material is normally found in considerable amount.

The experiments of this series show that the mature ovary furnishes a substance, presumably a hormone, controlling egg deposition. Furthermore, it seems that the source of the active principle is the follicular cell rather than the ovum itself: Extracts from freshly laid eggs or eggs just being extruded from the oviduct proved inactive.

(3) In order to test whether the "ovarian hormone" thus demonstrated acts on the oviduct directly, or via another gland of internal secretion, a third type of experiment was undertaken. Histophysiological evidence already discussed suggested a possible role of the neurosecretory cells of the protocerebrum. Therefore, clusters of neurosecretory cells from at least two donors whose pars intercerebralis contained neurosecretory material were transplanted into the prothorax of hosts which were not yet ready to deposit their eggs. The result was striking. Almost immediately the characteristic movements of the genital plates, the extension of the rostrum, and salivation could be observed. In eleven experimental animals oviposition started within 5 to 15 minutes. The implants of neurosecretory cells in these animals did not lead to a depletion of stainable material in their own pars intercerebralis.

The conclusion that neurosecretory material from the brain of *Iphita* furnishes a hormone inducing egg deposition is in line with the results obtained by ENDERS

(1955) who found an increase in the rhythmicity of the oviduct of *Carausius* following the administration of extracts from brains and corpora cardiaca.

A correlation of these experimental and histophysiological observations permits the following tentative conclusions (see Fig. 1). When containing mature eggs, the ovary releases into the hemolymph an active principle which acts on the neurosecretory cells of the pars intercerebralis. More specifically, this action seems to cause the release of neurosecretory material staining blue with GOMORI's method into the blood stream through the aortic wall in the region of the corpus cardiacum. An active principle present in this stainable material then causes the release of the eggs from the oviduct. Apparently, this takes place at a time when the corpus allatum does not receive neurosecretory material. Since this coincides with the period of temporary inactivity of this gland, preceding the onset of a new reproductive cycle, one may suggest that the neurosecretory material which, during the mating period, is seen to enter the corpus allatum may serve to activate it.

The results of this study may serve as an example to illustrate the existence of endocrine chain reactions in which neurosecretory centers play a decisive role (see B. SCHARRER, p. 79 of this Symposium).

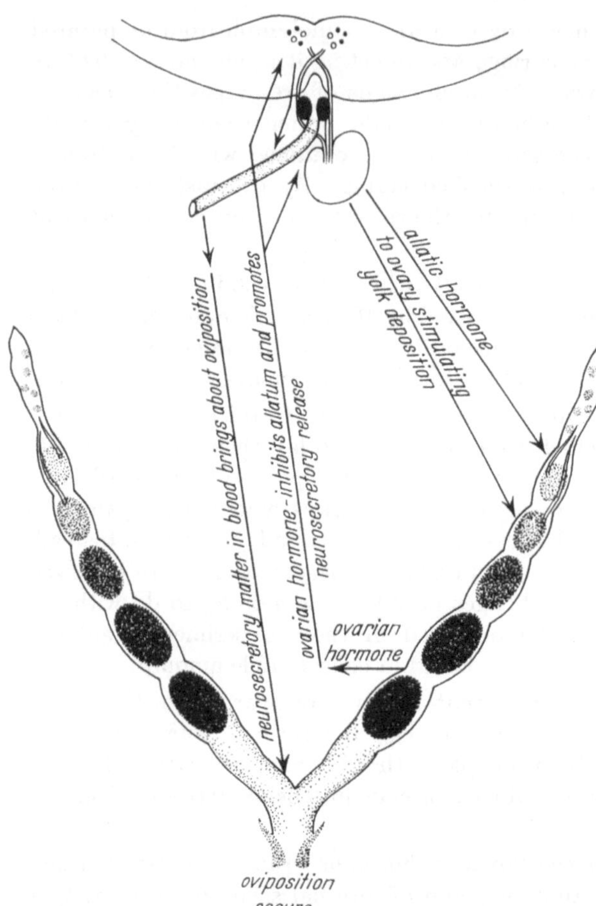

Fig. 1. Diagrammatic representation of the presumed interdependence of the reproductive organs and the neurosecretory system in the adult female of *Iphita limbata*. (1) The corpus allatum hormone stimulates yolk deposition in young eggs. (2) In the presence of mature eggs, the ovary releases a substance into the circulation. (3) This "ovarian hormone" stimulates the neurosecretory cells of the pars intercerebralis to release their contents into the aorta. The neurosecretory material released into the circulation brings about oviposition. The concomitant inactivation of the corpus allatum may be explained by its temporary lack of supply of neurosecretory material

References

DUPONT-RAABE, M.: Bull. Soc. zool. France **76**, 386—397 (1951).
— Arch. Zool. exp. gén. **89**, 128—138 (1952).
ENDERS, E.: Verh. dtsch. zool. Ges. Erlangen **1955**, 113—116.
SCHARRER, B.: The Hormones, Vol. III, p. 57—95. New York: Academic Press, 1955.

Marlborough College, Wiltshire, England

Electron Microscopy of a Crustacean Neurosecretory Organ

By

Francis G. W. Knowles

With 2 Figures

The term "neurosecretory" has been applied to those neurones in which considerable quantities of presumed secretory material can be demonstrated by simple histological means, and which do not apparently innervate any muscle or exocrine organ. Moreover it has been shown that many neurosecretory neurones contain physiologically active substances and that the spatial arrangement of these neurones indicates that their contained secretory products are released into the blood-stream and there act as hormones (6).

The sinus-glands, post-commissure organs and pericardial organs of crustaceans are neurosecretory organs within the terms of the above definition. They have been shown to consist principally of the terminations of fibres in which secretory material can be observed and from which active principles may be extracted. In addition to these undisputed neurosecretory organs other areas of the crustacean nervous system have been suspected of hormonal activity and it has been suggested that the three organs listed above are but some of the neurosecretory organs in crustaceans. In some instances claims for evidence of neurosecretion have been based on the observation of supposed secretory material but there has been no evidence that this material is released into the blood-stream (5). Clearly the presence of droplets or granules in neurones does not necessarily indicate neurosecretion, and it would be valuable to have further anatomical criteria to distinguish normal neurones from neurosecretory elements. The present study has been undertaken with the intention of determining whether, in addition to abundant secretory material, there may be other features which are characteristic of neurosecretory cells and which, though too small to be discerned through an optical microscope, might be revealed by the electron microscope. The work is still in progress and at this stage it is not possible to do more than indicate some interesting features in the structure of the neurosecretory fibres in the post-commissure organs of crustaceans.

The post-commissure organs of the Mediterranean crustacean *Squilla mantis* have been chosen for study because each of these organs is discrete and is easily removed without damage, is known to contain chromactivating substances, and is supplied by a relatively long nerve which may be easily sectioned (4). Thus far two principal areas have been studied (a) a proximal position of a post-commissure nerve, and (b) a portion of the neurohaemal release organ. The first contains mainly neurosecretory fibres; the second contains the terminations of these fibres. Since these terminations lie very close to the surface but some of the fibres of which they form a part are more deeply seated, some difficulty has been found in adjusting fixation to achieve an adequate and comparable electron density throughout. In these preliminary studies immersion in a 2% solution of osmium tetroxide in sea-water for five to ten minutes was found to be fairly satisfactory as a compromise between over-fixation of the surface areas and under-fixation of the inner regions (more recently I have found that longer periods of fixation, of 2—3 hours, give more consistently good results). After fixation the tissues were washed in mixtures of sea-water, tap-water and alcohol graduated so that the transference from the sea-water fixative to the solution of alcohol in tap-water was achieved with the minimum danger of osmotic change. The specimens were examined by the prototype model of the Metropolitan-Vickers E. M. 6 electron microscope, an E. M. 4 model and a Siemens Elmiskop 1.

Observations through the optical microscope had indicated that the neurosecretory fibres branch repeatedly as they near the post-commissure organs (3). Under the electron microscope it can be seen that before this branching takes place each fibre is surrounded by a multi-layered Schwann sheath, which appears to be spirally coiled, in a manner comparable to that which has been described for normal axons also (2). This sheath forms part of a Schwann or satellite cell, the nucleus of which is in many cases as large as or larger than the diameter of the fibre. Distal to the division of the fibre the fine fibres which result remain ensheathed by the multilayered sheath. The fibres begin to divide in the distal portion of the post-commissure nerve.

The inclusions in the axoplasm of fibres before and after division show interesting dissimilarities. Before division the axoplasm contains very numerous mitochondria, mostly arranged at the periphery directly beneath the axolemma, and surrounded by osmiophilic material (Fig. 1a). The presence of peripherally arranged mitochondria in crustacean axons has already been remarked (2) and so a comparison was made between the neurosecretory fibres in the post-commissure nerves and motor fibres innervating the mandibular muscles. It was found that the mitochondria of the neurosecretory fibres seemed to be at least five times more numerous and also larger than those in normal motor fibres. The abnormal number of mitochondria in the neurosecretory fibres indicates that considerable biochemical changes are taking place there, but it is impossible at present to tell whether these changes are involved in the manufacture of secretory materials or whether they are energising the passage of secretory material along the axons; possibly they may be actively engaged both in the production of material and in its transport.

Fibres in the distal portion of the post-commissure nerve contained few and relatively small mitochondria; a number of other inclusions which did not appear to be mitochondria, but which might be interpreted as secretory material, were seen. In some fibres many small granules were arranged round the periphery (Fig. 1b): In others small aggregates of material were seen (Fig. 2a).

In the post-commissure organs some neurosecretory fibres were very thin, little more than 1500 Å in diameter. A number of these seemed to approach

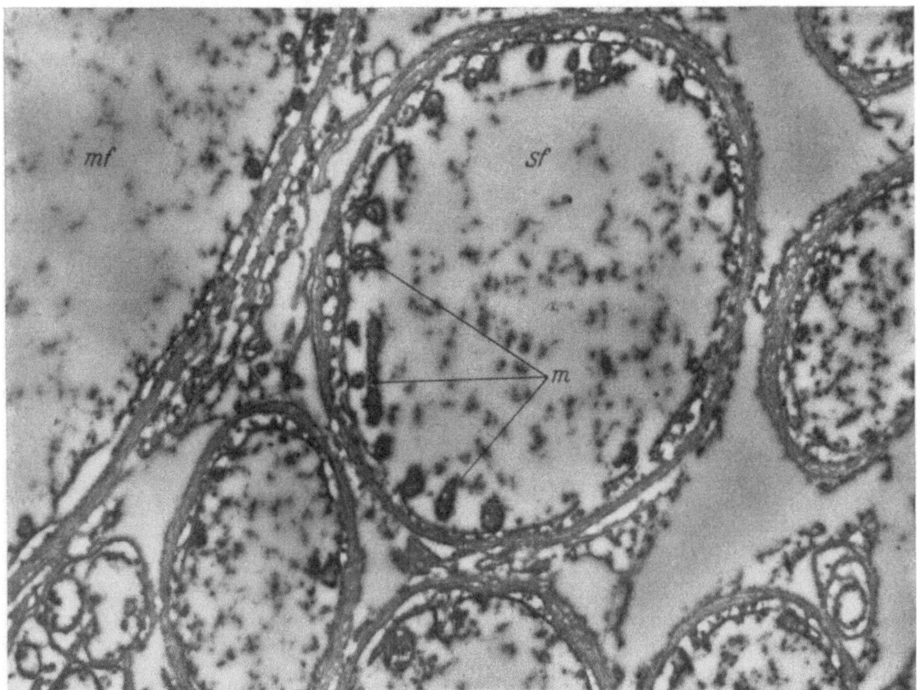

Fig. 1a. A motor fibre and some neurosecretory fibres in a post-commissure nerve of *Squilla mantis* in transverse section. *mf* Motor fibre; *sf* Neurosecretory fibre; *m* Mitochondria. Magnification 9,000 ×

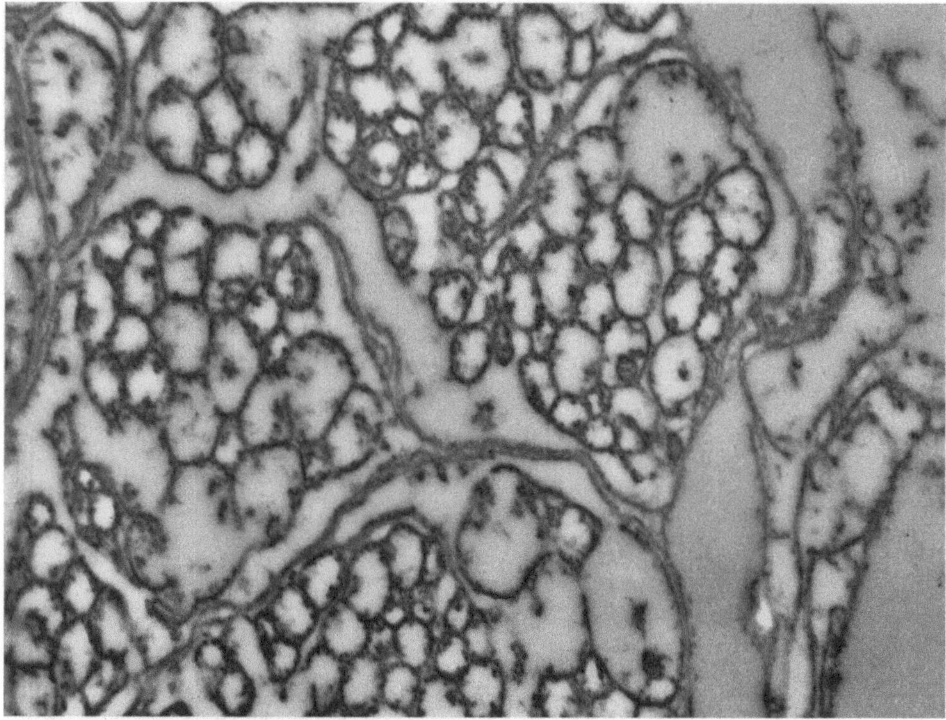

Fig. 1b. Some neurosecretory fibres in a post-commissure nerve of *Squilla mantis*. Each fibre contains some peripheral secretory droplets and occasional mitochondria can be seen. Each group of fibres represents the products of division of a fibre similar to that shown at plate 1a. Magnification 24,000 ×

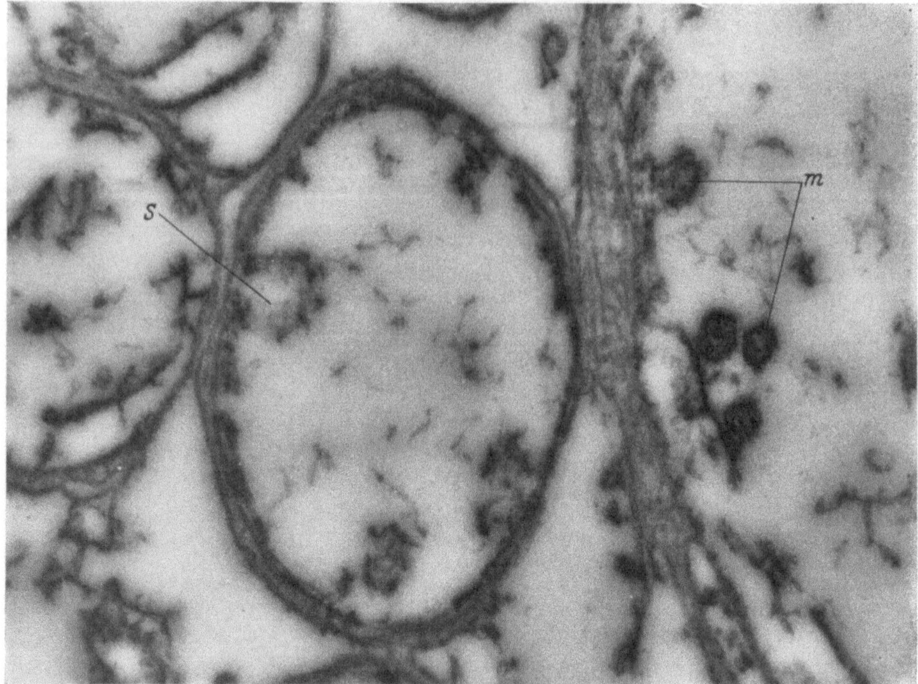

Fig. 2a. Neurosecretory fibres in transverse section. *s* possible secretory material; *m* Mitochondria.
Present Magnification 29,000 ×

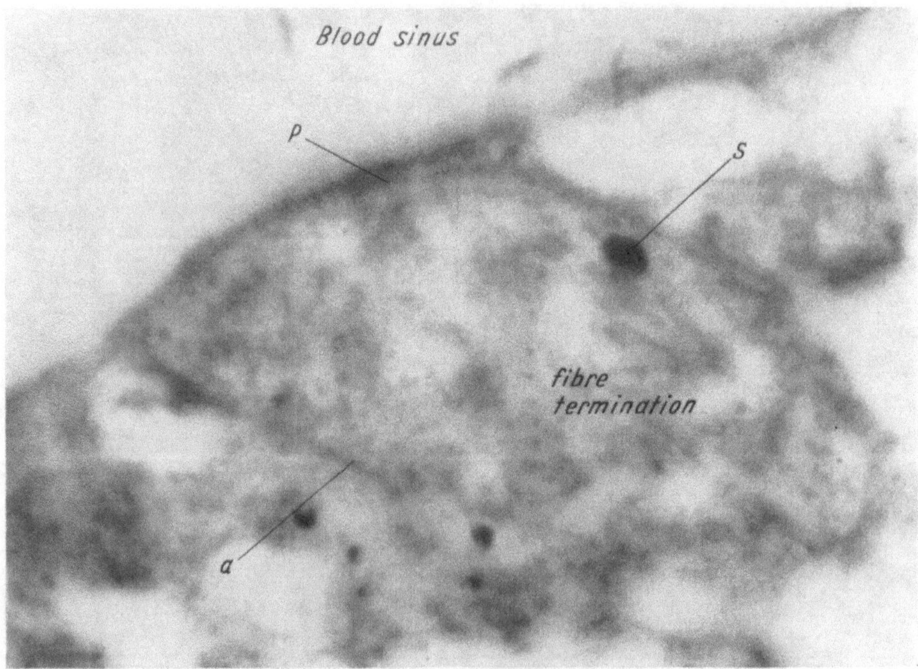

Fig. 2b. A longitudinal section through a termination of a neurosecretory fibre. *p* pore in axolemma
and basement membrane; *s* secretory material; *a* axolemma. Magnification 27,000 ×

the walls of blood-sinuses and then turn back, thus forming a loop directly beneath the blood-sinus membrane. At this point these fibres were still enclosed by the multi-layered Schwann sheath.

Finally the fibres terminated in bulbous endings, each about 1 micron in diameter, which lay in the epineurium, close to the blood-sinus basement membrane. At this stage the multi-layered Schwann sheath was no longer present (Fig. 2b). The fibre terminations contained some oval bodies about 1500 Å to 2000 Å in diameter.

Summary

Thus far the evidence from electron microscopy of the post-commissure organs indicates the possibility that secretory material may be manufactured by mitochondrial activity along the course of the fibres in each post-commissure nerve. When the neurosecretory fibres reach the neurohaemal release organ some form loops close beneath the surface of blood-sinuses, possibly to provide regions for storage of material [in this connection it is interesting to note that WINGSTRAND has described comparable loops in the hypothalamic-hypophysial tract in birds (7) and that BLISS and WELSH have remarked on the accumulation of secretory material in loops in the neurosecretory fibres leading to the sinus-glands of crabs (1)]. Finally the neurosecretory fibres appear to emerge from the Schwann cytoplasm which has hitherto enveloped them to terminate in swellings approximately 1 micron in diameter.

References

1. BLISS, D. E., and J. H. WELSH: Biol. Bull. 103, 157—169 (1952).
2. GEREN, B. B., and F. O. SCHMITT: Eighth Congress of Cell Biology, Leiden 1954.
3. KNOWLES, F. G. W.: Endeavour 14, 95 (1955).
4. — and D. B. CARLISLE: Biol. Rev. 31, 393—473 (1956).
5. MATSUMOTO, K.: Biol. J. Okayama Univ. 1, 234—238 (1954).
6. SCHARRER, E., et al.: Pubb. Staz. Zool. Nap. 24. Suppl. (1954).
7. WINGSTRAND, K. G.: The structure and development of the avian pituitary. Lund: Gleerup 1951.

Reed College, Portland, Oregon, USA

Neurosecretion and Retinal Pigment Movement in Crustaceans

By

L. H. KLEINHOLZ

Retinal and integumentary pigment cells are two types of crustacean effectors known to be hormonally influenced by a neurosecretory product from the eyestalks. Initial studies by HANSTRÖM (1937) and subsequently by BROWN (1940) indicated that the sinus gland is probably the major source of chromatophore-activating substances in the crustacean eyestalk, but later investigators [BLISS, DURAND and WELSH (1954), KNOWLES (1953), POTTER (1954)] showed histologically that a complex neurosecretory network exists in the crustacean central nervous system and that major pathways of this network from the ventral nerve cord and optic ganglia terminate in the sinus gland. The sinus gland thus appears to consist largely of the secretion-laden endings of neurones whose cell bodies might be located at some distance from the sinus gland itself. A series of tests by injection experiments supplied additional evidence that chromatophore-activating substances were present in the combined or separated optic ganglia of the eyestalk and in the ventral nerve cord as well as in the sinus gland [BOWMAN (1949), BROWN (1950), SANDEEN (1950)].

Two questions in this area of crustacean endocrinology have persisted for a long time with only meager experimental information: 1) the localization of origin of the retinal pigment hormone, and 2) the identity or non-identity of the retinal pigment and chromatophore-activating hormones. This note reports the results of some studies directed toward these two questions. The portion of the study concerned with retinal pigment activity of neurosecretory material from *Pandalus* and *Calocaris* was done in collaboration with Dr. D. B. CARLISLE at the Kristineberg Marine Station in Sweden.

The localization experiments consisted of comparisons between the effects of injections of extracts prepared from whole eyestalks on the distal retinal pigment of the dark-adapted test animals *(Palaemonetes vulgaris* and *Leander adspersus)* and the effects of extracts, similarly prepared, of components of the eyestalk and central nervous system (i. e., sinus glands, medulla terminalis and other ganglia of the eyestalk, thoracic ganglia, and ventral nerve cord). The standardized testing procedure was to inject 0.05 ml. of extract of tissue from the donor species into the dark-adapted test species and then to measure the amount of movement of the distal retinal pigment toward the light-adapted position at intervals of 30—45 minutes after injection; extracts of whole eyestalks and of the separated components were prepared in similar concentrations, generally 10 per ml.

It became apparent from such experiments that striking differences existed between the retinal pigment activity of components of the brachyuran eyestalk and of the macruran eyestalk. Extracts of sinus glands from brachyurans showed little or no retinal pigment activity as contrasted with extracts of the sinus-glandless eyestalk or of separated ganglionic components of the eyestalk. On the other hand, similarly prepared extracts from the eyestalks of macrurans showed retinal pigment activity to be almost as high in the sinus gland as in the entire eyestalk. The results of such comparative studies are summarized in Table 1.

Table 1. *Responses of the distal retinal pigment of two test species. Palaemonetes vulgaris and Leander adspersus were injected with extracts of neurosecretory tissue. In all cases but Callinectes sapidus, where the concentration of the extracts was 6 units per ml., the concentration of the extracted tissue was 10 units per 1.0 ml. Injections were made into dark-adapted test animals and the position of the distal retinal pigment measured 30—45 min. after the injection; the position of the pigment in the uninjected controls shows the pigment position in the dark-adapted retina and increase in the numerical value for this position represents a proximal migration of the distal pigment toward the light-adapted position.*

Donor species	Tissue extract	Average position of distal pigment in microns
A. Palaemonetes vulgaris as the test animal		
Carcinus maenas:	whole eyestalk	229
	sinus gland	86
	eyestalk minus sinus gland	210
	medulla terminalis	92
	control (uninjected)	55
Libinia emarginata:	whole eyestalk	217
	sinus gland	132
	eyestalk minus sinus gland	197
	thoracic ganglia	123
	control (uninjected)	58
Callinectes sapidus:	whole eyestalk	225
	sinus gland	81
	eyestalk minus sinus gland	213
	control (uninjected)	59
B. Leander adspersus as the test animal		
Pandalus borealis:	whole eyestalk	253
	sinus gland	279
	eyestalk minus sinus gland	226
	purified erythrophore hormone preparation of ÖSTLUND and FÄNGE	59
	control (tissue extract injection)	60
	control (uninjected)	41
Nephrops norvegicus	sinus gland	251
	eyestalk minus sinus gland	210
	control (uninjected)	36
Calocaris macandreae:	protocerebrum and optic stalk including sinus glands	45
	control (uninjected)	34

In an approach to the second question mentioned above, the action of known chromatophore-activating substances was tested on the distal retinal pigment. A highly-purified hormone preparation of ÖSTLUND and FÄNGE (1956), known to cause blanching of erythrophores in *Leander adspersus* (1 mg. of this preparation contains about 10 million *Leander* units) caused only very slight movement of the distal retinal pigment in this prawn. Extracts of the protocerebrum and optic lobes (including the sinus glands) of *Calocaris macandreae*, a blind prawn, were without effect on the distal retinal pigment of *Leander* when concentrations as high as 80 per ml. were tested, although concentrations of 10 per ml. caused blanching of dispersed erythrophores.

These observations indicate the possibility of striking differences in the neurosecretory regulatory mechanisms for the distal retinal pigments of brachyuran and macruran crustaceans. They also indicate a separation of the hormones acting on the two major types of pigmentary effectors, chromatophores and retinal pigment.

Literature

BLISS, D. E., J. B. DURAND and J. H. WELSH: Neurosecretory system in decapod Crustacea. Z. Zellforsch. **39**, 520—536 (1954).
— and J. H. WELSH: The neurosecretory system of brachyuran Crustacea. Biol. Bull. **103**, 157—169 (1952).
BOWMAN, T. E.: Chromatophorotropins in the central nervous organs of the crab,*Hemigrapsus oregonensis*. Biol. Bull. **96**, 238—245 (1949).
BROWN, F. A JR.: The crustacean sinus gland and chromatophore activation. Physiol. Zool. **13**, 343—355 (1940).
— Studies on the physiology of *Uca* red chromatophores. Biol. Bull. **98**, 218—226 (1950).
HANSTRÖM, B.: Die Sinusdrüse und der hormonal bedingte Farbwechsel der Crustaceen. Kgl. Svensk. Vetenskapsakad. Handl. **16**, 1—99 (1937).
KNOWLES, F. G. W.: Endocrine activity in the crustacean nervous system. Proc. roy. Soc. London B **141**, 248—267 (1953).
ÖSTLUND, E., and R. FÄNGE: On the nature of the eye-stalk hormone which causes concentration of the red pigment in shrimps (Natantia). Ann. sciences naturelles Zool. et Biol. anim. **18**, 325—334 (1956).
POTTER, D. D.: Histology of the neurosecretory system of the blue crab, *Callinectes sapidus*. Anat. Rec. **120**, 716 (1954).
SANDEEN, M. I.: Chromatophorotropins in the central nervous system of *Uca pugilator* with special reference to their origins and actions. Physiol. Zool. **23**, 337—352 (1950).

Biological Laboratories, Harvard University, Cambridge, Mass., USA

Observations on the Neurosecretory System of Portunid Crabs*

By

David D. Potter

With 4 Figures

A study has been made of the inclusions found in living and fixed nerve cells in the central nervous systems of two genera of portunid crabs, *Callinectes* and *Carcinus*. In order to discover if any of the types of inclusions found in neurosecretory cells is unique to these cells, and therefore, by inference, directly associated with the production, transport or storage of hormonally active substances, the inclusions of nerve cells whose endocrine function is not in doubt have been compared with inclusions of other nerve cells in the eyestalk, brain and thoracic ganglion.

Living neurosecretory cells of the X organ-sinus gland complex (Fig. 1) contain three classes of inclusions, distinct in size, optical properties and staining properties. All can be found in the cell bodies of the medulla terminalis X organ, in the axons of the sinus gland nerve and in the nerve terminals of the sinus gland (Fig. 2). The smallest of these inclusions are the most interesting. They are 0.1—$0.3\,\mu$ in diameter, have a slightly lower refractive index than their surroundings and do not stain with Janus green, methylene blue or neutral red. They are responsible for the characteristic blue-white color of the living neurosecretory cells under dark field illumination. They are almost certainly homologous to the basic secretory granules described by Passano (1954). These fine particles fill the nerve terminals in the sinus gland as sand fills a sand bag, and within a single terminal or fiber they are uniform in size. Near their

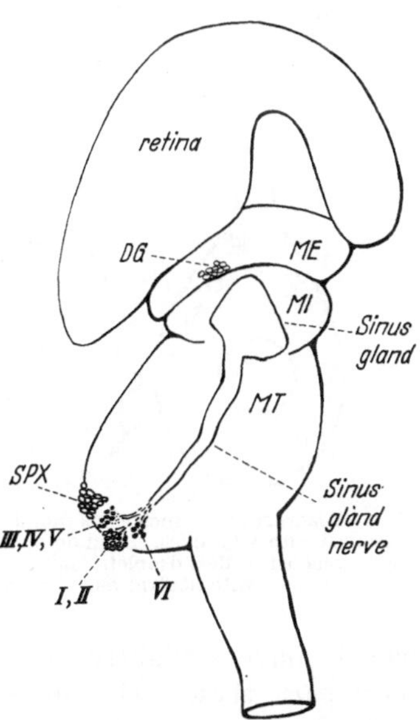

Fig. 1. Diagrammatic dorsal view of the ganglia of the right eyestalk of *Callinectes*. The ventral part of the medulla terminalis (*MT*) has been pulled anteriorly to show the *X* organ. *DG* dorsal group of nerve cells (see text). *ME* medulla externa; *MI* medulla interna; *SPX* sensory pore *X* organ. The Roman numerals indicate the types of neurosecretory cells found within the three groups of nerve cells which comprise the medulla terminalis *X* organ

* An abstract of part of a thesis presented to Harvard University in partial fulfilment of the requirements for the degree of Doctor of Philosophy. This work was supported in part by an E. L. Mark Fellowship and in part by a National Science Foundation Predoctoral Fellowship.

terminals the thin-walled neurosecretory fibers often possess very large, and almost certainly temporary, swellings which may be considered modifications for storage of the fine particles.

The second class of inclusions presumably consists of mitochondria. These bodies are 0.4—0.7 μ in diameter, have a high refractive index and stain selectively with Janus green. They are not uncommon in sinus gland nerve endings. The third class of inclusions is more heterogeneous than the first two. It includes bodies 1.0—5.0 μ in diameter which stain selectively with neutral red and which

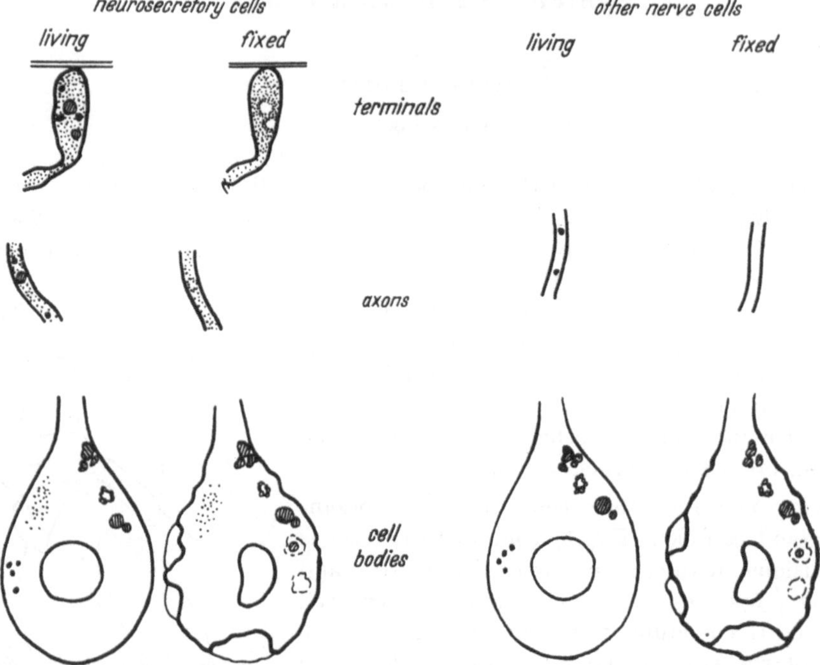

Fig. 2. Diagram of the inclusions found in crab nerve cells. Stippling: fine particles, 0.1—0.3 micron in diameter, unstained with vital dyes. Solid dots: mitochondria, 0.4—0.7 micron in diameter, selectively stained with Janus green. Shaded bodies: droplets, flakes and clusters of granules, 1.0—5.0 microns in diameter, selectively stained with neutral red. Unstained vacuoles occur in fixed but not in living nerve cells

usually have a slightly higher refractive index than their surroundings. For the most part, these inclusions look and behave like emulsified oil droplets. Some, at least, are artifacts, for their numbers increase as living preparations age. In the cell bodies, inclusions in this size range may also appear flake-like or they may consist of a cluster of granules of mitochondrion-size.

At one time or another, most types of nerve cells of the central nervous system (Fig. 2), from the smallest cells to the largest motor cells, contain each of these types of inclusions, except the fine particles. The fine particles have been found only in the neurosecretory cells of the X organ-sinus gland complex and in two other very restricted cell groups, one near the sinus gland (Fig. 1, DG), the other in the thoracic ganglion. Their restricted occurrence, intracellular distribution, small size and large numbers suggest that these fine particles are associated in some way with the active substances known to be produced by X organ neurosecretory cells [Bliss (1953), Passano (1953)]. The neutral red-stained droplets, on the other hand, have a very general distribution in crab nerve cells and presumably have a very general function. They strikingly resemble the lipochondria described in crustacean nerve cells by Parameswaran (1956), in molluscan nerve cells by many workers [see Chou (1957), for references] and in insect nerve cells by Shafiq (1953), Shafiq and Casselman (1954), Nayar (1955) and Malhotra (1956). The fine particles may prove to be a useful criterion for distinguishing neurosecretory cells from other nerve cells, if it can

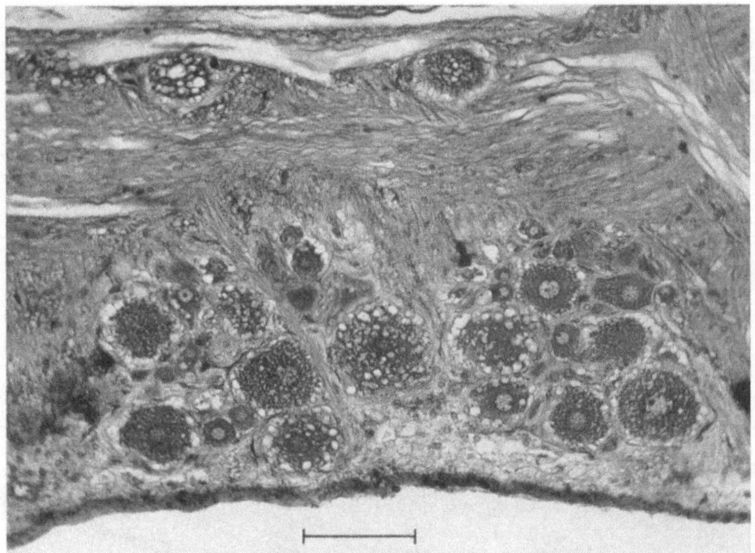

Fig. 3. Large motor cells in a Bouin-fixed thoracic ganglion of *Callinectes*.
Many cells contain vacuoles which have no visible counterparts in living cells. Scale: 100 microns

be demonstrated that the hormonal activity of the eyestalk neurosecretory system is, indeed, associated with a particulate fraction of this size.

In ordinary histological preparations, both the fine particles and the larger droplets can be identified. The staining properties of the fine particles are discussed below. At least certain of the neutral red-stained droplets are represented in histological preparations by droplets which stain with azocarmine, phloxine, acid fuchsin, or, under certain circumstances, with aldehyde fuchsin. The difference between the fine particles and the droplets is usually as striking in fixed cells as in living cells, especially in tissues fixed in osmium tetroxide and stained with azan. In the latter, the fine particles are stained with azocarmine, to the exclusion of almost every other structure in the eyestalk, and the droplets are simply darkened with osmium.

Fixed nerve cells frequently contain not only the particles and droplets described above but also inclusions which do not have visible counterparts in carefully handled living cells. The most common of these are unstained vacuoles (Fig. 3) which may occur singly or in great numbers in a single cell. It has been observed that vacuoles can be produced by the action of fixatives on living cells.

The variety of staining reactions shown by the fine particles is a striking feature of the crab X organ-sinus gland complex. This has been described by a number of workers [see review by KNOWLES and CARLISLE (1956)], most of whom have interpreted the varied staining reactions as an indication that there is a chemical transformation of a secretory product. However, in certain portunid crabs it is clear that there are at least six distinct tinctorial types of fine particles in the sinus gland, produced by six distinct types of neurosecretory cells in the medulla terminalis X organ. The six types of fine particles are readily demons-

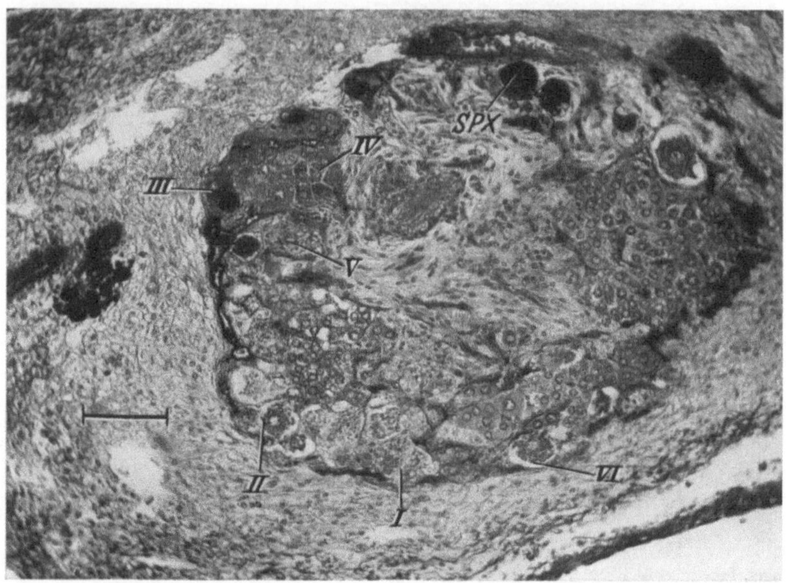

Fig. 4. Oblique section through the *X* organ region of a *Callinectes* eyestalk which was fixed in Bouin and stained with azan. Roman numerals indicate the positions of the six types of neurosecretory cells. *SPX*: element of the sensory pore *X* organ. Scale: 100 microns

trated in preparations fixed in Bouin and stained with Heidenhain's Azan or with DAWSON's (1953) or ROSA's (1953) aldehyde fuchsin techniques. Since particular endocrine functions cannot yet be assigned to any of these cells, the neurosecretory cells are arbitrarily designated Types I—VI. The common staining reactions of the fine particles in these types of cells are summarized in Table 1. No single dye has been found which stains all the fine particles, nor does any of the dyes used stain only the fine particles.

The most convincing evidence that the six tinctorial reactions are neither random artifacts nor the result of chemical transformations of less than six types of fine particles is the fact that each tinctorial type of fine particle is seen to arise in nerve cell bodies which have a characteristic location and distinctive morphology (illustrated in part in Figs. 1, 4). Additional evidence for the distinctiveness of the six cell types is provided by the following facts.

1) Type III cells differ from all the others in that they are invariably found in much larger numbers in female crabs than in male crabs (Table 1).

2) Type IV cells differ from all the others in that they are smaller and in that they are the only cells containing fine particles which stain strongly with aldehyde fuchsin with Rosa's technique.

3) Types V and VI differ from the others in that their endings in the sinus gland are invariably localized in the region near the point of entry of the sinus gland nerve.

4) Within a single fiber there is no change in the staining reaction of the fine particles for as far as the fiber can be followed, often more than three-quarters of its length.

5) The color of the fine particles within a cell body, axon, or ending is not related to the number of the fine particles.

Table 1. *Neurosecretory cells of the X organ-sinus gland complex in Bouin-fixed eyestalks of adult Callinectes sapidus*

Cell Type	Dye which stains the fine particles	Approx. cell diameter	Approx. number of cells	Approx. % of endings in the sinus gland
I	azocarmine (red)	50 microns	100	females: 60 males: 75
II	orange G (yellow)	50 microns	20	10
III	azocarmine and aniline blue (purple)	60 microns	females: 60 males: 2 ?	females: 20—25 males: 1 ?
IV	aldehyde fuchsin (purple)	15 microns	25	5
V	orange G (orange)	20 microns	females: 8 males: 11	5—10
VI	aniline blue (blue)	30 microns	6	5—10

6) There is an obvious tendency for all the sinus gland endings of a given color to be filled with, or emptied of, fine particles synchronously.

7) When a large number of sinus glands is examined it is obvious that the number of fine particles of any one color varies independently of the number of fine particles of any other color.

8) There are constant differences between species in the proportion of the sinus gland which is made up of endings of a given color. It is interesting that in such distantly related species as the grapsoid crab *Ocypode* and the oxystomatous crab *Calappa* cells can be found in the medulla terminalis X organ which correspond precisely in location and staining reaction to neurosecretory cells in the X organ of *Callinectes* and *Carcinides*.

Nothing has been seen which suggests that the sinus gland contains endogenous secretory cells.

Under certain circumstances, axons containing fine particles which show Type I and Type II staining reactions can be found in the optic lobe peduncle. Type II axons have also been seen in the circumesophageal connectives, and cell bodies containing Type II fine particles have been found in one restricted location in the thoracic ganglion.

These observations provide a morphological basis for the endocrinological complexity of the crab eyestalk [KNOWLES and CARLISLE (1956)].

Bibliography

BLISS, D. E.: Endocrine control of metabolism in the land crab, *Gecarcinus lateralis* (Freminville). I. Differences in the respiratory metabolism of sinusglandless and eyestalkless crabs. Biol. Bull. **104**, 275—296 (1953).

CHOU, J. T. Y.: The cytoplasmic inclusions of the neurones of *Helix aspersa* and *Limnea stagnalis*. Quart. J. Micr. Sci. **98**, 47—58 (1957).

DAWSON, A. B.: Evidence for the termination of neurosecretory fibers within the pars intermedia of the hypophysis of the frog, *Rana pipiens*. Anat. Rec. **115**, 63—69 (1953).

KNOWLES, F. G. W., and D. B. CARLISLE: Endocrine control in the Crustacea. Biol. Rev. **31**, 396—473 (1956).

MALHOTRA, S. K.: The cytoplasmic inclusions of the neurones of certain insects. Quart. J. Micr. Sci. **97**, 177—186 (1956).

NAYAR, K. K.: Studies on the neurosecretory system of *Iphita limbata* Stal. I. Distribution and structure of the neurosecretory cells of the nerve ring. Biol. Bull. **108**, 296—307 (1955).

PARAMESWARAN, R.: Neurosecretory cells of the central nervous system of the crab, *Paratelphusa hydrodromous*. Quart. J. Micr. Sci. **97**, 75—82 (1956).

PASSANO, L. M.: Neurosecretory control of molting in crabs by the X-organ sinus gland complex. Physiol. Comp. Oecol. **3**, 155—189 (1953).

— Phase microscopic observations of the neurosecretory product of the crustacean X-organ. Pubbl. Staz. zool. Napoli **24**, 72—73 (1954).

ROSA, C. G.: Preparation and use of aldehyde fuchsin stain in the dry form. Stain Tech. **28**, 299—302 (1953).

SHAFIQ, S. A.: Cytological studies of the neurones of *Locusta migratoria*. Part I. Cytoplasmic inclusions of the motor neurones of the adult. Quart. J. Micr. Sci. **94**, 319—328 (1953).

— and W. G. B. CASSELMAN: Cytological studies of the neurones of *Locusta migratoria*. Part III. Histochemical investigations of the neurones with special reference to the lipochondria. Quart. J. Micr. Sci. **95**, 315—320 (1954).

Isolation of the Red Pigment Concentrating Hormone of the Crustacean Eyestalk

By

PEHR EDMAN*, RAGNAR FÄNGE** and ERIC ÖSTLUND***

With 1 Figure

Among the substances probably produced by neurosecretory cells are the colour change hormones or chromatophorotropins in crustaceans. Several such hormones acting on red, black and white chromatophores have been demonstrated, but the exact number is not agreed on. The first one discovered was the hormone causing concentration of red chromatophores in prawns and occurring mainly in the sinus gland of the eyestalk. Since the discovery of this hormone a number of others have been described, and several workers have tried to isolate and chemically define various colour change hormones.

CARSTAM (1936) summarized the known chemical and physical properties of the red-pigment-concentrating hormone, which at that time was not clearly distinguished from other eyestalk principles. ABRAMOWITZ (1940) prepared colour change hormone from eyestalks of *Uca* by methods which are used for the isolation of nitrogenous bases. His preparations were bioassayed on black chromatophores of *Uca*, but they also affected red pigment in *Palaemonetes*. BROWN and SCUDAMORE (1940) compared the effect of extracts of eyestalks from different species on black chromatophores in *Uca* with that on red pigment in *Palaemonetes*. Their results indicated that the effects were due to two different hormones, one dispersing the black pigment and the other concentrating the red one. BROWN and KLOTZ (1947) investigated a pigment-concentrating substance in the central nervous system of *Crangon*. They found the substance soluble in ethyl, methyl and isopropyl alcohol. FINGERMAN (1956) showed that in the crab *Callinectes* the red-pigment-concentrating principles of the sinus gland and of the circumoesophageal connectives were both soluble in ethanol in contrast to the hormone which disperses the black pigment.

KNOWLES, CARLISLE and DUPONT-RAABE (1955) used paper electrophoresis to study chromatophorotropins from crustaceans and insects. In sinus glands, post-commissure organs and corpora cardiaca they found a red-pigment-concentrating substance probably of peptide nature. In addition they described a number of other substances with similar actions. In an electrophoretic study of sinus gland extracts from *Uca*, STEPHENS, FRIEDL and GUTTMAN (1956) found that a substance with red pigment concentrating activity moved as a single peak.

A large scale preparation of the red-pigment-concentrating hormone in eyestalks was made by ÖSTLUND and FÄNGE (1956). Adsorption on a column of

* Institute of Medical Chemistry, University of Lund, Sweden.
** Department of Zoophysiology, University of Lund.
*** St. Erik's Hospital, Medical Department, Stockholm.

aluminum oxide yielded a highly purified preparation. Further results from this work will be presented in this article.

Material

Our source for the preparation of the hormone, as in the previous work by Östlund and Fänge (1956), consisted of eyestalks from *Pandalus borealis*. This shrimp species is commercially caught along the Swedish West coast and is very abundant. The suitability of this material as a source of hormone for chemical studies was first realized by Carstam (1951). The hormone preparations were assayed on specimens of the prawn, *Leander adspersus*. An arbitrary unit of hormone activity was defined by Östlund and Fänge (1956). The hormone concentration in the different steps of the purification process has been measured in this unit.

Method of Purification

Eyestalks (several kg) were extracted with acetone. After filtration the acetone was evaporated off. The watery residue was washed with ether in order to remove inactive fat-soluble substances. After concentration to dryness in vacuo the remainder was treated with boiling ethanol. This treatment precipitates proteins not removed by acetone and dissolves the hormone. The ethanol extract, after concentration in vacuo, was redissolved

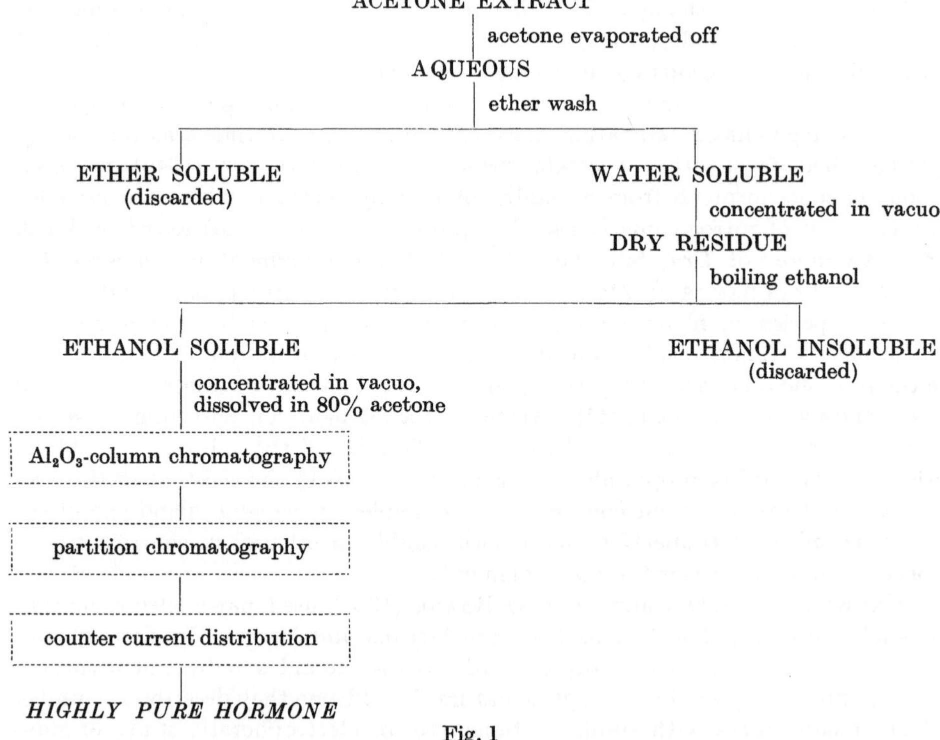

Fig. 1

in a few ml of 80% acetone. Adsorption on a column of aluminum oxide according to Östlund and Fänge (1956) followed. The hormone was eluted from the column with 70—80% acetone. This acetone extract was concentrated to a tar-like residue, which had a biological activity of about 100000 units/mg. (We have estimated the hormone content of a single eyestalk to be 3000 units; the weight of an eyestalk is about 40 mg.). The hormone preparation still contained considerable impurities such as UV-fluorescent substances, brown pigments and inorganic salts. For further purification we used methods which were based on the specific solubility properties of the red pigment-concentrating hormone, i. e. partition chromatography and Craig counter current distribution. The characteristic properties of the hormone in different solvents were studied in preliminary experiments.

The partition chromatography was performed on a column of silica (Hyflo supercel) using as a solvent a water-saturated 1 : 1 mixture of n-butanol and amyl alcohol. About 100 consecutive fractions were collected. The most active fractions were pooled and concentrated by evaporation in vacuo.

For further purification the counter current distribution principle was utilized. The two solvents consisted of a buffer solution (p_H 2.4) and a 1 : 1 micture of n-butanol and ether. The active fractions from the counter current distribution were pooled and concentrated in vacuo to dryness. The final product was some 30—40 mg of a slightly brownish coloured, somewhat sticky substance.

A scheme of the purification procedure is given in Fig. 1. The experimental details of the partition chromatography and of the counter current distribution technique are to be described in a later publication.

Chemical Properties of the Purified Hormone

Solubility in different solvents. In agreement with several previous investigators we have found that the hormone is easily soluble in ethanol and other low-molecular alcohols, but nearly insoluble in non-polar organic compounds. Table 1 shows some results from studies of the partition of the hormone between

Table 1. *Partition of the hormone between organic solvents (organic phase) and buffer solutions (inorganic phase)*

	Ethyl acetate		n-Butanol		Dichloro-ethylene		Cyclohexane		Ether	
p_H	2.5	9.5	2.5	9.5	2.5	9.5	2.5	9.5	2.5	9.5
Activity in org. phase . . .	*	0	***	***	0	0	0	0	*	0
Activity in inorg. phase . .	***	***	0	*	***	***	***	**	***	***

Number of stars indicate degree of activity. Zero sign indicates no activity.

a water phase and a variety of organic solvents. It is seen that the hormone is somewhat soluble in non-polar solvents (ethyl acetate, ether) at low p_H but not at high p_H.

Paper chromatography. An R_f-value of 0.43 was found for the purified hormone when a water-saturated mixture of n-butanol and amyl alcohol was used as solvent. Localization of the hormone in the chromatograms was made exclusively by bioassay. No chemical reaction was found by which the hormone could be identified. The ninhydrin reaction was negative and so was the peptide reaction of REINDEL and HOPPE (1954). Negative results were also obtained with Pauly's and Ehrlich's reagents and with the iodine azide reaction for sulfur.

Paper electrophoresis. These experiments were performed in buffer solutions of p_H 2.5, 4.0, 7.0 or 9.0. Thiophenylurea was used as an uncharged reference substance. After completion of the electrophoresis (about 12 hours; 300 V) strips of the dried filter paper were assayed for their biological activity. It was found in all cases that the hormone moved slightly towards the anode, the movement being somewhat more pronounced at high p_H than at low p_H.

Inactivation by enzymes. 200000 units of the hormone were completely inactivated in 1 minute by a 1 : 1000 solution of chymotrypsin (Table 2). Inactivation of the same amount of hormone could also be obtained with a 1 : 1000 solution of crystalline trypsine after incubation for 6 hours at 36° C.

Acid hydrolysis. The purified hormone was remarkably stable both in acid and alkaline dilute solutions. Heating for 6 hours at 100° in 6-N hydrochloric acid completely abolished the activity. Samples from this hydrolyzed preparation were investigated by paper chromatography which showed the presence of at least 4 amino acids. At present we have no proof that these amino acids were obtained from the hormone rather than from impurities.

Table 2. *Inactivation by chymotrypsin* (p_H 7.8; temp. 18° C; 200,000 units of purified hormone)

Enzyme conc. (gms/ml)	Inactivation time (minutes)
5×10^{-5}	206
10^{-4}	60
5×10^{-4}	23
10^{-3}	1

Biological Activity

When assayed on *Leander adspersus* the purified hormone had a biological activity of about 10000000 units/mg dry weight. As yet no other biological effects than the concentration of red chromatophores have been observed. The red-pigment-concentrating effect has been found in several species of Natantia: *Leander adspersus, L. squilla, L. serratus* and *Lysmata seticaudata.* Experiments with crabs *(Carcinides maenas)* showed that in these animals amputation of the eyestalks caused a dispersion of red pigment. Injection of the purified hormone in eyestalkless crabs had a concentrating effect upon the red pigment. No effects were seen on the black or white pigments in *Leander* and *Carcinides.* The dark pigment in the chromatophores of the isopod *Idothea baltica* was not affected by the hormone.

During the biological experiments it was repeatedly observed that following injection of large amounts of the hormone (about 1000 units) into eyestalkless specimens of *Leander adspersus* a "blue reaction" occurred. This phenomenon, which has been observed by several previous investigators, seems to be a transformation of red pigment into a blue forming a halo around the red chromatophores. However, the true nature of the "blue reaction" ought to be more closely studied.

Conclusions

The eyestalks of *Pandalus* contain a red-pigment-concentrating substance with an extremely high biological activity. The hormone is inactivated by chymotrypsin, trypsin and by prolonged treatment with strong hydrochloric acid. It may be a polypeptide, but definite proof of this is still lacking. According to the electrophoresis experiments it has an acid character. The increased solubility in ether and ethyl acetate at low p_H also indicates that it has acid properties.

In the experiment with crabs no black-pigment-dispersing effect was noticed. Thus by the preparation method used the red-pigment-concentrating hormone seems to have been completely separated from the black-pigment-dispersing substance also occurring in the eyestalk. However, the two hormones possibly belong to the same category of substances, because the black-pigment-dispersing hormone is also inactivated by chymotrypsin [WELSH (1957)].

By the isolation method described the hormone causing concentration of red pigment may be obtained in a very pure form.

References

ABRAMOWITZ, A. A.: Purification of the chromatophorotropic hormone of the crustacean eyestalk. J. biol. Chem. **132**, 501—506 (1940).

BROWN, F. A. JR., and I. M. KLOTZ: Separation of two mutually antagonistic chromatophorotropins from the tritocerebral commissure of *Crago*. Proc. Soc. exp. Biol. (N. Y.) **64**, 310—313 (1947).

— and H. H. SCUDAMORE: Differentiation of two principles from the crustacean sinus gland. J. cell. comp. Physiol. **15**, 103—119 (1940).

CARSTAM, S. P.: Color changes in brachyuran crustaceans, especially in *Uca pugilator*. Kgl. fysiogr. Sällsk. Lund Förhandl. **6**, 63—80 (1936).

— Enzymatic Inactivation of the pigment hormone of the crustacean sinus gland. Nature (Lond.) **167**, 321 (1951).

FINGERMAN, M.: Black pigment concentrating factor in the fiddler crab. Science **123**, 585 to 586 (1956).

KNOWLES, F. G., D. CARLISLE and M. DUPONT-RAABE: Studies on pigment-activating substances in animals. I. The separation by paper electrophoresis of chromactivating substances in arthropods. J. Mar. biol. Ass. U. K. **34**, 611—636 (1955).

ÖSTLUND, E., and R. FÄNGE: On the nature of the eye-stalk hormone which causes concentration of red pigment in shrimps (Natantia). Ann. Sci. nat. Zool. 11e sér. **18**, 325—334 (1956).

REINDEL, F., und W. HOPPE: Über eine Färbemethode zum Anfärben von Aminosäuren, Peptiden und Proteinen auf Papierchromatogrammen und Papierelektrogrammen. Chem. Ber. **87**, 1103 (1954).

STEPHENS, G. S., F. FRIEDL and B. GUTTMAN: Electrophoretic separation of ·chromatophorotropic principles of the fiddler crab, *Uca*. Biol. Bull. **111**, 312—313 (1956).

WELSH, J. H.: Personal communication.

Summary

The concept of neurosecretion as it emerged from the discussions of the Naples Symposium has proved fruitful in many ways; it served once more as the basis of the agenda of the Lund Symposium. The neurosecretory cell may still be defined as a nerve cell which receives nervous impulses, but does not pass them on to other neurons or effector organs. The axon of the neurosecretory cell ends at the wall of a blood space into which it releases its product. It is, of course, conceivable that a neuron discharges visible secretory granules anywhere on its surface, while its axon maintains synaptic connections with other cells. However, no such case is known at present, and the definition of the neurosecretory cell as a nerve cell which secretes microscopically demonstrable granules via its axon into the blood is still valid.

The results of electron microscopy studies reported at the Symposium confirm with an added measure of precision earlier findings obtained by light microscopy. The stainable neurosecretory material as seen in the light microscope after the conventional treatment of fixation, embedding and staining appears to result from clumping of submicroscopic granules of a rather uniform size which seems characteristic for each species. These granules are always observed within the perikaryon, the axon, and the terminal axonal swelling; they do not lie outside on the surface of the cell and they do not occur in ordinary nerve cells.

Earlier ideas concerning the constituents of these granules have proved correct, at least with respect to the neurosecretory material of the hypothalamic-neurohypophyseal system of pig and cattle. It appears now well documented that physiologically active polypeptides are attached to large protein molecules representing the stainable component (neurophysin). In view of the variety of neurosecretory systems in invertebrates and vertebrates a great deal of chemical research will be required before the composition and significance of neurosecretory products is adequately understood.

There are reasons to believe that, in the case of the hypothalamic-pituitary neurosecretory system of the vertebrates, polypeptides other than oxytocin and vasopressin may be attached to the protein molecule. These polypeptides may play a role in the release of anterior lobe hormones such as ACTH. These and similar agents await identification.

It becomes increasingly evident that the production by neurosecretory cells of hormones such as oxytocin and vasopressin is only one and perhaps a less important aspect of neurosecretion. As more and more neuro-endocrine systems are being studied, the role of the neurosecretory cell as mediator between nervous system and endocrine system becomes increasingly evident. The endocrine system can no longer be considered as a closed system whose constituents control each other exclusively by feedback mechanisms. Actually, both hormonal and nervous factors may well act through the central nervous system in which all incoming messages can be integrated to act on one common final pathway controlling production and release of a particular hormone. It now appears that the neurosecretory cell is the common final pathway for the transmission of messages to organs of internal secretion. The recognition of the importance of the neurosecretory cell as a link in neuro-endocrine pathways may well lead to a better understanding of these pathways.

Thus, the neurosecretory cell is no longer an oddity of doubtful significance. Largely as a result of the Naples Symposium it has become more generally recognized as a special cell type. It may be predicted that the Symposium at Lund will help to speed up the investigation of neuro-endocrine systems which depend on neurosecretory cells for the integration and transmission of impulses from the nervous system to endocrine organs. The exploration of these neuro-endocrine relationships in invertebrates and vertebrates constitutes a large field of research. We may look forward to an exciting third symposium on neurosecretion sometime in the future.

Teilnehmerverzeichnis

Dr. R. Acher, Laboratoire de Chimie Biologique de la Faculté des Sciences, Place Victor Hugo, Marseille/France

Prof. W. Bargmann, Anatomisches Institut der Universität Kiel/Deutschland

Dr. (and Mrs.) D. B. Carlisle, The Laboratory, Citadel Hill, Plymouth/England

Dr. Jakob Christ, Max-Planck-Institut für Hirnforschung, Gießen/Deutschland

Dr. Marie Dupont-Raabe, Laboratoire de Zoologie, 1 Rue Victor Cousin, Paris/France

Fil. mag. Anders Enemar, Zoologiska Institutionen, Lund/Sverige

Prof. U. S. von Euler, Fysiologiska Institutionen, Stockholm 60/Sverige Solnavägen 1

Fil. mag. Gunnar Fridberg, Zootomiska Institutet, Rådmansgatan 70 A, Stockholm Va/Sverige

Dozent Ragnar Fänge, Zoofysiologiska Institutionen, Lund/Sverige

Prof. (and Mrs.) Bertil Hanström, Zoologiska Institutionen, Lund/Sverige

Dr. C. L'Hélias, Laboratoire de génétique évolutive, Gif sur Yvette/France

Dr. (and Mrs.) Arne S. Johansson, Zoologisk Laboratorium, Blindern, Oslo/Norwegen

Dr. P. Karlson, Max-Planck-Institut für Biochemie, Goethestr. 31, München 15/Deutschland

Dr. Lewis Kleinholz, Reed College, Portland 2, Oregon/USA

Sir Francis Knowles, Marlborough College, Wiltshire/England

Dr. H. Legait, Dr. E. Legait, Laboratoire d'histologie de la Faculté de Médecine, Nancy/France

Dr. P. O. Lundberg, Anatomiska Institutionen, Uppsala/Sverige

Dr. Bruno Malandra, Istituto di Anatomia Patologica, Università di Pavia, Via Forlanini 14, Pavia/Italia

Dr. Luciano Martini, Via A. Del Sarto 21, Milano/Italia

Prof. Valdo Mazzi, Istituto di Anatomia Comparata, Via Giolitti 34, Torino/Italia

Fil. mag. Claes von Mecklenburg, Zoologiska Institutionen, Lund/Sverige

Fil. mag. Patrick Meurling, Zoologiska Institutionen, Lund/Sverige

Fil. mag. Ragnar Olsson, Zootomiska Institutet, Rådmansgatan 70 A, Stockholm Va/Sverige

Dr. E. Östlund, Fysiologiska Institutionen, Karolinska Institutet, Stockholm/Sverige

Dr. Bernard Possompès, Conférences de Biologie Animale, Sorbonne, Paris (5e)/France

Dr. (and Mrs.) David D. Potter, Biophysics Department, University College, Gower Street, London W. C. 1/England

Dr. Alan B. Rothballer, Albert Einstein College of Medicine, 1300 Morris Park Avenue, New York 61/USA

Dr. (and Mrs.) M. Saffran, Allan Memorial Institute, McGill University, Montreal/Canada

Prof. Yutaka Sano, Department of Anatomy, College of Medicine, Kamikyoku, Kyoto/Japan

Dr. Berta Scharrer, Prof. Ernst Scharrer, Albert Einstein College of Medicine, 1300 Morris Park Avenue, New York 61/USA

Dozent Th. H. Schiebler, Neue Universität, Haus 30, Anatomisches Institut Kiel/Deutschland

Dr. J. C. Sloper, Department of Morbid Anatomy, Charing Cross Hospital Medical School, 62, Chandos Place, London W. C. 2/England

Dr. Fred Stutinsky, 12 Rue Cuvier, Paris (5e)/France

Prof. (and Mrs.) Paavo Suomalainen, Universitetets Zoologiska Laboratorium, Rautatiekatu 13, Helsinki/Suomi-Finland

Dr. Ellen Thomsen, Prof. Mathias Thomsen, Den Kgl. Veterinaerhøjskole, Bülowsvej 13, København/Danmark

Prof. John H. Welsh, Biological Laboratories, 16, Divinity Ave., Cambridge 38, Mass./USA

Prof. V. B. Wigglesworth, Department of Zoology, Downing St., Cambridge/England

Prof. Karl Georg Wingstrand, Universitetsparken, 3, København Ö/Danmark